YOUR WIFE HAS CANCER...

now what?

Published by Familius LLC, www.familius.com
Familius books are available at special discounts for bulk purchases for
sales promotions, family, or corporate use. Special editions, including
personalized covers, excerpts of existing books, or books with corporate logos, can be created in large quantities for special needs. For more
information, contact Premium Sales at 801-552-7298 or email special-
markets@familius.com

Library of Congress Catalog-in-Publication Data

2013933823

pISBN 978-1-938301-42-1
eISBN 978-1-938301-41-4

Physical book printed in the United States of America
Book design by Kathryn Brinton and David Miles
Photography by Carson Boss
Cover design by David Miles
Edited by Tammy Simpson

10 9 8 7 6 5 4 3 2 1

First Edition

YOUR WIFE HAS CANCER...

now what?

*What to expect when the
unexpected happens.*

CARSON BOSS

Contents

Endorsement

A diagnosis of cancer can be devastating physically, emotionally, and financially. This is even truer when the diagnosis is given to the love of your life. As a surgeon who deals with this diagnosis on a daily basis, I believe providing the patient and her family with as much information as possible is an important first step on the potentially long road to survivorship. My patients are my heroes with their courage and strength.

Many of my patients are supported by wonderful husbands/partners. Much like parenting though, many husbands have a steep learning curve during this stressful period. In this book, Carson provides a guide for husbands/partners of cancer patients, kind of a "What to expect when the unexpected happens." This book is a must read for any husband hoping to shorten their learning curve.

I highly recommend it.

Leigh Neumayer, MD, MS
Professor of Surgery
Co-Director, Multidisciplinary Breast Cancer Program
Huntsman Cancer Institute
University of Utah

Preface

When your wife is diagnosed with cancer there is *a lot* of information provided. You might get overwhelmed with the number of pamphlets, books, and binders that discuss her particular type of cancer. She will find information on dozens of support groups, hotlines, and other organizations to assist her.

But what about husbands?

When I looked for guidance in the materials we were given, I noticed a web chat link and a hotline number for concerned loved ones to get help and suggestions, but nothing specific for me as her husband. So I began a process of reaching out to husbands I knew whose wives had cancer and found their insight and advice to be priceless.

Their experiences, coupled with my own, brought me to the realization that we all shared similar experiences, no matter what type of cancer our wives had.

For all of the lost husbands who do not know what to do, this book is for you!

Even though there are many scientific studies and lengthier books available, my intent is to give you information that's to the point, along with a practical outline that addresses thirteen common areas. Also included is a checklist so you can make notes and customize your own action plan.

To help your wife fight this, you will need all the assistance you can get.

This may be her battle, but you are her soldier!

Acknowledgments

First and foremost, I would love to tell Cindy, my beautiful wife and companion, how fortunate I feel to have her in my life. Talk about a pillar of strength. Through it all she kept our family functioning on all cylinders. Her encouragement and undying devotion to our four wonderful children and me have given us a blueprint on the proper way to live our lives during difficult times. Ask anyone who has come in contact with her and they will always mention her smile, her laugh, her warmth, and the genuine love she demonstrates. Thanks for all the strength and courage you have shown and continue to show battling through this.

I would like to tell Cody, McKinley, Keaton, and Parker how proud I am to be their father and thank them for the support they gave Mom. They made sure to watch each other and their friends for signs of illness. They became masters of disinfectant wipes. Whenever they were sick, they would offer to stay at Grandma's until they got better so they would not contaminate their mother. They did their best to give her the space she needed, while she was healing or after treatments. They sure grew up quickly with the added responsibility, but it has given them new understanding about forgetting oneself and putting the needs of others above your own.

To my parents, Paul and Paula, and my in-laws, Brent and LaRene, without whom my family would've been woefully short-handed, thank you. You showed genuine love with all of the meals, sleepovers, housework, and shuttling children. This includes my wife's grandparents and our brothers, sisters, aunts, uncles, cousins, nieces, and nephews. Thanks so much for all of your help and prayers which were truly answered.

I would like to mention a few of the couples that were an example of how my wife and I could get through it together: Kevin and Nikki Johnson, Matt and Shea Saylor, Lynn and Judy Boss, Terry and Kay Alger, Steve and Tanna Coleman, Brad and Denise Morris, Kent and Rochelle Godfrey, Paul and Debbie Widdison, and Larry and Claudia Kirby. I would also like to mention the great couples that I've met through the "Young Survivors Sister Group." There are also many other friends and neighbors that shared their experiences, tragedies, and triumphs that helped me realize we are all on this journey of life together, and the more we help each other the easier it can be.

A special thanks to Dr. Leigh Neumayer, Dr. Jayant Agarwal, Dr. Sheila Garvey, Dr. Harold Johnson, Dr. Robert Harris, and Dr. Larry Smithing. To you and all of your staff of nurses and technicians . . . you really took care of my wife and made sure we were comfortable every step of the way.

CHAPTER ONE

Experience with Cancer

Most of us have had experience with cancer in our past. Whether it was with family members or mere acquaintances, we probably knew about cancer and what it can do as a disease. As the following timeline will show, I was aware of cancer at various times in my life.

TIMELINE

"Your Grandma Has Cancer"

I was seven years old when my parents told me my paternal grandmother had a cancerous brain tumor that had come back after an earlier surgery to remove one that was benign. Due to complications from this second surgery, she spent the remaining months of her life in a nursing home.

Visiting her in that condition was a terrible experience. She was my caregiver a few days per week while both of my parents were at work. I could not understand why she would not wake up and recognize me anymore. I wanted to still be by her side cracking a big bowl of peanuts while watching the children's shows on TV.

She was the first person that I was close to that had died from cancer and even though I was very young, it had a profound effect on me. The word "cancer" had the ability to take someone I love away from me.

"Your Grandpa Has Cancer"

I was twenty-three years old when my mother informed me that my maternal grandfather had lymphoma cancer that had spread to his liver. He went through chemotherapy and was able to prolong his life another couple of years from these treatments.

It was tough to see a man who was very strong and had a very intense work ethic shrink down to half his size and not have the energy to do more than a few dishes here and there. The loss of weight and the change in appearance were very evident and alarming to me.

I felt very fortunate, however, that these treatments allowed him to be there for my wedding when he was supposed to have passed away before that time.

"Your Grandmother Has Cancer"

I was thirty-one when my mother informed me that my maternal grandmother had been diagnosed with breast cancer. She had a mastectomy, with no recurrence. but did not need any other treatments.

This was my first experience with someone having the mastectomy procedure and she chose not to do reconstruction nor wear prosthesis. Let's just say that I noticed this every time I hugged her and it took a while to get used to.

"Your Sister Has Cancer"

I was thirty-six when my mother informed me that my sister had cancer. She went through some painful surgeries and treatments for two different types of cancer without recurrence. It started with what she thought was a canker sore on her tongue that wouldn't heal. It turned out to be mouth cancer that they would find out later had spread to her thyroid.

Up to this point in my life, cancer had affected my grandparents only so I had come to the conclusion that my parents might have to deal with it next. I was totally unprepared to see this happen to my older sister. She was the one that was the best babysitter I had ever had, the one that would make my favorite kind of cookie, and the one who had blessed my life with five nephews and one niece. It was a real gut check to realize it could happen to anyone at any age.

"Your Wife Has Cancer!"

I was coming up on my fortieth birthday when this statement changed everything for me. I was not prepared to hear this. Who is? That statement kept repeating over and over in my mind. Although I had experienced this disease through close members of my family, I was not prepared to think of these words in relation to the woman that had been by my side for seventeen years and the mother of our four young children.

So how did we get to that point?

OUR STORY

It was about a week after Christmas when my wife called me into the bathroom and mentioned she had found a small lump on her breast. She asked me what I thought. She had mentioned that her breasts were unusually tender after her most recent menstrual cycle and she was just checking her breasts when she noticed the lump.

There Is No Such Thing as a Good Lump

All lumps are abnormalities and should not be there.

In this age of increasing cancer risk, I was glad my wife was aware of the change in her body. She thought it might be a cyst at first, but this did not feel soft like a common cyst. It was round and hard. She continued to suggest that maybe it was a clogged or infected pore, but the surrounding area was not red.

These suggestions just didn't add up and the lump alarmed us both . . . with good reason.

Many of my wife's relatives on her dad's side had dealt with different types of cancer. Like me, my wife had experience with this disease while growing up. Due to her family's history, she already had several mammogram screenings. The screening from a year prior had been clean, so she really wasn't worried at this time. I told her to make an appointment with her OB/GYN as soon as possible to get the lump checked. She then scheduled another mammogram and the report was sent directly to her doctor.

My wife's doctor called with concerns about the results of the report. His wife had battled through breast cancer, so my wife could sense the urgency in his voice. He recommended her to the cancer specialist that was in his clinic.

On to the Specialist

My wife's first attempt to make an appointment was unacceptable, at least in my opinion. The doctor's office was scheduled a few weeks out, so she just took the first one available. My wife can be timid and accommodating sometimes, so I told her to call them back and mention her family's history with cancer . . . or I would. She did and they were able to get her in that week.

I could really feel my wife's apprehension during the visit with the cancer specialist. She had a hard enough time getting used to her OB/GYN, let alone having other doctors look at personal areas of her body. It was also hard for me to see my wife examined. I tried to keep the mood as light as I could by asking questions and making small talk, not only for my wife's sake, but for mine as well. After she was examined, the specialist confirmed that she did not like the hardness of the lump and that my wife should have a biopsy. The specialist did mention however, that the majority of the lumps tested come back non-cancerous. This felt reassuring initially, but we still remained anxious.

The Biopsy

My wife and I went over to pathology where they performed what is called a Punch Biopsy. The ultrasound technician finds the lump while another technician uses a tool that has a circular blade that is rotated down through the skin and into the lump to get a three to four millimeter cylindrical core tissue sample (you will get used to talking medical as well). He was able to get some good samples through the initial incision that looked like very small worms. It amazed me that something so small could possibly have such grave consequences depending upon the results of their testing.

Our hope and prayer from the biopsy was that no matter what the results were, we wanted a definitive answer as to whether or not it was cancerous. We did not want to hear that they were not quite sure and would need further testing. If the biopsy was inconclusive, a surgical procedure called a lumpectomy would have to be performed in order to determine whether or not the lump was cancerous.

The Results

A few days later, my wife and I went back for the results of the biopsy. Talk about the longest five-day wait of our lives. Even more painful was the wait for our specialist to come and go over the biopsy results. When the specialist came in, there was no small talk and she got right to the point.

"The biopsy results came back cancerous!"

At first I was a little angry at such a quick comment, since I don't think anyone is ever prepared to hear those words. Where was the small talk or the build up? But in hindsight, I'm glad she didn't sugarcoat the news or beat around the bush. I figure it is less painful to rip the band-aid off in one quick motion than gradually tear it off bit by bit.

I will never forget the glance my wife and I shared at that moment. It almost seemed surreal, like we were suspended in a dream that we would wake up from at any minute. But unfortunately it wasn't a dream.

Now What?

Much to my wife's credit, she kept it together and simply asked the doctor, "Now what?"

The doctor immediately went into how it was a common form of breast cancer called Invasive Ductal Carcinoma (IDC). The cancer was treatable, but my wife would need to get some more tests which included blood work, another ultrasound, chest x-rays, a Magnetic Resonance Image (MRI), and some genetic testing called the BRCA testing. All of these would aid in finding out what stage of cancer she had so a treatment plan could be developed. As hectic as it was for her to get all of this done, it was overwhelming for me to try to wrap my mind around these foreign terms and pro-cedures. The bottom line in my mind was, "She has cancer and nothing can change that now!"

This Was Only the Beginning

I had always been an outside observer when dealing with this disease in my family. The reality of their cancer had never been in the forefront of my mind. I would only think about it when I received updates from other family members or while making visits. Other priorities of my life would soon take over and my accountability to them would end.

Now it was on me.

As her husband, I could not pawn responsibilities off on others. I was about to be involved in ways I could never imagine.

My journey was just beginning!

CHAPTER TWO

Shock and Fear

*To describe all of my feelings when my wife was diag-
nosed would take a lot of time to explain. My life quickly
became an emotional extreme roller coaster. However, there
were two main emotions that emerged simultaneously . . .
shock and fear. Other husbands concurred that these were
predominant with them as well.*

I had experienced shock and fear individually at different
times throughout my life, but rarely at the same time. I can
instantly recall where I was and what I was doing when
Mount St. Helens erupted or when I witnessed the live feed
of the Challenger space shuttle disaster or the images of the
terrorist-hijacked planes crashing into the Twin Towers before my eyes. It shocked me that these events could happen.

The fear would soon settle in with the realization of how little control I have in this world . . . outside of myself.

THE PATTERN

Finding out my wife had cancer brought these two emotions of shock and fear front and center. The shock that this could happen to such a healthy person was followed by the unrelenting fear of losing her.

Based on my previous experience with cancer, I figured it was a disease you get when you're older or have lived a good long life. The shock was my wife having cancer in her thirties and the fear of not knowing what it was doing to her body. There was definitely a repetitive thought pattern that left me feeling helpless.

Question after question kept flooding my mind. What stage was her cancer? What's the survival rate of each stage? What are the treatments and side effects? What happens if it has spread? What would happen to the children and me if we lost her? How would I raise four young children by myself???? One dark thought after another kept piling up and consuming my thoughts.

SLEEP DEPRIVATION

Sleep became difficult for me after the diagnosis. I would wake up time after time just staring at my wife with my mind racing. I knew it was taking a toll on my health and I needed to pull myself out of this rut.

But how?

I walked around in a daze until I finally made the decision to deal with the reality of the situation. I had to come to the realization that people do die from cancer . . . but the majority of those diagnosed survive. I needed to change my outlook to get out of the fog I was in.

To help quell these emotions, I went back to those world events I mentioned earlier and realized if I could get through those, then I could get through this. Up to this point they were the most notable experiences I had in overcoming these two emotions, but now it was more personal. Mount St. Helens was replanted, space missions continued on, New York City and the nation moved on. No matter the outcome with my wife's cancer, I had to believe I could accept it and move forward.

FAITH

My religion and belief in God were also paramount in helping me deal with these emotions. I came to realize that life offers the good with the bad, and we have to learn to "manage" both. Granted, matters of life and death can be more ominous, and this was definitely one of those times. Still, you have to decide that you will fight these feelings so you can help your wife fight these same emotions as well.

The husbands I reached out to commented that thei⸱ faith in a higher power helped them as well. Some were able to overcome these emotions quickl⸱

others took longer. No two people are alike, but they all learned to keep their belief and let it carry them through.

Once I was able to get on top of my feelings of shock and fear, I had to get answers to the questions that were constantly going around in my mind. You have to be able to keep your head clear so you can learn as much as possible about your wife's type of cancer.

CHAPTER THREE

Knowledge Is Power

Once you know what type of cancer you are dealing with, what the test results are, and how to manage your emotions, you will be able to find answers to the questions that have been weighing on your mind.

I had never studied any one cancer in detail. I was amazed at all of the types that women can get and how common they are.

Here's a statistical reference in order of their prevalence:

- All types of cancer (1 in 3)
- Breast cancer (1 in 8)
- Lung and bronchus (1 in 16)
- Colorectal (1 in 20)
- Uterine corpus (1 in 39)

- Non-Hodgkin lymphoma (1 in 52)
- Melanoma of the skin (1 in 55)
- Urinary bladder (1 in 87)
- Leukemia (1 in 91)
- Uterine cervix (1 in 147)

Rebecca Siegel, MPH; Elizabeth Ward, PhD; Otis Brawley, MD; Ahmedin Jemal, DVM, PhD, "Cancer Statistics, 2011," CA: A Cancer Journal for Clinicians 61, no. 4 (2011): onlinelibrary.wiley.com/doi/10.3322/caac.20121/pdf.

ONE IN THREE

The statistic that really caught my attention was the first one. One in three women will get some form of cancer in their lifetime. I had no idea it was that common.

I never got into the root causes and treatment options of my extended family members who had cancer. I left that up to my parents, who would take them to their appointments and therapies. Because I wasn't a medical student and lacked intimate experiences caring for a loved one, my only references were the worst-case scenarios that I had seen on television or in the movies. I developed an extreme sense of foreboding with the term cancer.

THE INTERNET

It became my obsession to learn as much as I could about Invasive Ductal Carcinoma. When my wife's biopsy information came back, I was able to take those findings and type them directly into a search engine where links to dozens of websites popped up. I was so thankful for modern technology. I can't imagine finding out my wife had cancer thirty years ago, which would mean having to rely on outdated medical pamphlets or visiting the local library, hoping they had enough information to appease me. Can you imagine trudging through large medical books, with even larger medical terms, trying to find out about one of the over two hundred different types of cancer?

The Internet was my saving grace.

In a matter of hours, I had learned so much about this specific type of cancer, and it was explained in terms I could actually understand. It was also comforting to go from one website to another and find consistency. You want to know the information you are getting has been verified by different sources and having them just a click away was especially helpful.

INFORMATION OVERLOAD

Your wife's focus may be different from yours. Some family and friends will join you on this path of acquiring knowledge and learn everything they can. Other people might not care to know the specifics and just focus on getting the patient well. Either way, *you* will have to be the encyclopedia.

I can't tell you how many times my wife asked me the same question again and again about something I had studied. She relied on me to help her remember what had been learned and what the terminology meant. Spending a few hours learning the terms will also make your doctor's visits more effective. Asking the right questions will produce the answers you need. Knowledge will give you a tremendous sense of empowerment.

CREDIBLE INFORMATION

As you begin your quest for knowledge, you will notice some websites are easier to read and navigate while others have more reliable information than others. By reliable I mean that some go into greater detail about the history, research, and studies than others. You might be perfectly happy in getting the basic information from some sites, but I preferred to go a little deeper into the background of breast cancer studies and treatment evolution. Some of my favorite websites, which contain good information for husbands and caregiver family members, are listed below along with the reasons why I like them.

- American Cancer Society (www.cancer.org): One of the oldest cancer organizations so they know how to explain the information you need. Easy to use layout with a nice Caregivers Section tab with good information on what you can do to help.
- Huntsman Cancer Institute (www.huntsmancancer.org): Another easy to use website with a great Patient-Family Support tab and good guidance.
- Cancer Treatment Centers of America (www.cancercenter.com): Simple format and easy to use tabs to access information on different types of cancer.

- Mayo Clinic (www.mayoclinic.com): Great site with historical information and how cancer treatments have evolved over time.
- Web MD (www.webmd.com): Effective job of touching on cancer advancements from the major cancer institutes around the world. Also, a good family medical reference.

CHAPTER 4

Getting the Word Out

Getting the word out can be tedious, so break it into sections.

You will need to adapt the information to different people in your relationship circle. Some will want to know everything and others will want just the basics, so be prepared for both.

CHILDREN

If you have more than one child, you will be dealing with different maturity levels. My children ranged in age from six to twelve, and I was worried how they would handle the news. The majority of counsel I received from other fathers was to explain it to the children in a direct manner, and then deal with their individual reactions. Do not assume how they are going to react or try to hide information from them. You might make matters worse.

We decided to present the information to our children together. We first asked them what they knew about cancer. Then, each one explained what they had heard or been taught about the disease. I was surprised how informed our two oldest were. We talked about other people they knew who had it. Letting them realize for themselves that it is a common disease helped cushion the blow when we told them about their mom.

Our oldest three children took the news rather well, at least initially. They asked a few questions, and because I had studied up on her type of cancer beforehand, I was able to customize the information into age appropriate terms. However, our six-year-old began to cry, saying he didn't want his mom to lose her hair. He had a dream several months before the diagnosis that his mom was bald and he could see the veins in her head, which was the basis for his fear.

Be Prepared

Although the children's initial reaction might seem well received, each child will process the news differently. Be prepared to handle different behavioral issues that might present themselves later on. These were some of the reactions I noticed:

- Trouble concentrating in school/drop in grades

- Acting out more than usual
- Increased arguing with parents and others
- Increased dependency on your wife
- An unusual desire to remain home with your wife

Our children exhibited many different emotions in the first few months.

Our oldest son was cruising through his first year of junior high school with decent grades, but they soon began to drop after the diagnosis. He admitted that his mind would wonder during class about what was happening at home. By the time he regained his focus in class, he would be behind in the discussion or miss taking down important notes. He also became a little more impatient with his younger brothers, due to the fact that they were together more than usual while we were away at all of the doctor appointments. He had to become the default babysitter quite a bit and it took him a while to get used to that role and responsibility.

Our daughter became very nurturing of my wife during the day, but would get possessive of her at bedtime. She really wanted her there to talk to at night and had a hard time sharing her mom with her brothers. She became more of a homebody and a little more closed off socially from her friends. There might have been some embarrassment with the sympathy she would receive from her friends and teachers.

Our youngest two sons bickered a little more than usual, trying to vie for their mother's attention. They also would sleep over at their grandparents more readily than before due to the changes at home in regards to their mother. Even though we did our best to act as normal as possible, those first few months I think they could sense the apprehension we felt with the unknown and what was coming.

As time passed, however, the children found various personal ways of coping. For example, when my wife lost her hair from chemotherapy, it became a nightly ritual for them to kiss her head before bedtime. It seemed to be their way of embracing the situation and losing their fear. They also became used to the additional attention and inquiries they would get in regards to their mom's health. They learned a lot about breast cancer and could answer people with great detail.

Sometimes you might not see a return to normal behavior patterns, which means they continue to struggle with it. Just know there are counseling options available if you feel your children's reactions and emotions are beyond your ability to help. You might not have the open communication kind of relationship, so a family therapist might be useful.

Teachers and Counselors Need to Know

It is also important to let your children's teachers and school counselors know what is going on so they can inform you if they notice any of the above reactions or other unusual behavior. For instance, when our oldest son's grades really took a nosedive the first quarter after the diagnosis, it was good for him to meet with the school counselor and realize that his lack of concentration was normal, and they could help him work through it.

Your children may miss school due to medical circumstances, so an open dialogue with their teachers is paramount. However, if you can help them keep regular attendance at school and a consistent routine, it will be to their advantage. This will help them pull out of the initial shock quicker.

Adult Children

For children not living at home, you might feel the need to hold back certain details thinking they have their own busy lives to worry about. It is important to be as up front with them as possible. You could be more technical with the diagnosis than you are with younger children still living at home.

A common reaction for adult-age children is they might want to spend more time with your wife, so don't be surprised to have a full house again. A few of the husbands I talked to told me their unmarried adult children practically moved back in, which is understandable. The married children with children of their own also increased their visits, which felt, at times, like they moved back in as well. Just be patient and let them deal with it in their own way.

But, here's a warning!

If you notice these constant visits and the increased commotion stressing your wife out, you will need to step in. She will not tell the children and grandchildren that they are negatively affecting her. Let your children know that she needs her rest to recover and schedule their visits when she's less vulnerable to fatigue.

HER PARENTS

The earlier you inform your wife's parents the better. My wife told her mother about her lump when she first noticed it, but wanted to wait to tell her father until she knew what her diagnosis was, so he didn't have to worry.

This was not the best course of action.

If he had known about the lump initially, I think it would have helped to temper his shock. This is hindsight, of course. Making the call to her parents to tell them their daughter has cancer was too big of a bomb to drop without a buffer period for him to get his emotions together.

How her parents react to this news is totally unpredictable. You did not grow up with them, and you probably have limited experience with how they act in stressful situations. Most likely they will feel helpless and will want to be more involved in your life. You might feel inundated with all of the calls you will receive, but understand their position. She is their daughter and they will be as scared as anyone. I had to keep reminding myself that if it were my daughter going through this, I would want to know all the details and how I could help.

You will need to exhibit patience as you explain the same information multiple times. Their concentration level will be interrupted by extreme emotions, as well as making it difficult for them to remember everything you are saying.

Give Them Accurate Information

Make sure you relay information to them as you receive it from the doctor so they know exactly what you know. You do not want them calling the doctors directly because you are not giving them enough information! This will only frustrate you and her doctors.

If you are fortunate enough to have a great relationship with your in-laws, embrace their interest and accept their help where possible. This can strengthen your bond with them. The sooner you subdue any ego of trying to do every-thing on your own, the easier it will be on all of you.

If you don't have a great relationship, do the best you can. Communicate through email or have one of your chil-dren relay information for you. Do not put it on your wife to deal solely with her parents. She needs to focus on her health, not on what her parents are going through.

YOUR PARENTS

Like your in-laws, the sooner your parents know the better. They can also be a great help. My parents offered to take the children during surgeries and treatments, so my in-laws and I could be there for my wife. I was glad they relied di-rectly on me for information and contacted her only when she felt up to it.

FRIENDS & NEIGHBORS

Some men are more outgoing than others. But no matter what personality extreme you gravitate to, you need to get the word out to others as soon as possible . . . with your wife's blessing, of course. You need to let her decide what information she wants to have shared.

Some husbands will hop on Facebook, Twitter, or other chat rooms and tell the world about their wife's cancer. Do not do this without clearing it with her first!

Once you have the green light and know exactly what she wants to share with others, it's good to tell your closest friends, neighbors, co-workers, and then your social media contacts. You will be amazed at the support you will receive, as cancer has touched everyone's life in some way. People will try to relate to your situation by recalling their own experiences. Even though no one can truly understand exactly what you both are going through, they can offer empathy and support. This will really help you.

While some people will jump in and offer to help, others might have a more difficult time and withdraw for a while. Understand it can be hard for some to share their emotions.

Do not pick and choose who to tell and who not to tell. Excluding certain people can lead to awkward feelings in the future. For instance, I had failed to make sure some of my close friends from high school knew about my wife's cancer. We went to see one of them in a play. When we went up to congratulate him on his performance, he didn't even recognize her. She was in the midst of chemotherapy and her appearance had totally changed. Needless to say, he felt like he had ignored her and was very embarrassed that he didn't know about her cancer. He would've made a point of her well-being and given her a hug. I felt awful about him not knowing.

Do Not Change

Even though your wife's cancer will change you, it is important to maintain your relationship with your friends. It can be difficult with all of the added responsibilities and pressures you will deal with, but if you totally withdraw from them, it will be hard to get some of them back. You do not want friends to disappear from your life. Relying on them will bring comfort and strength.

If you have activities that you do with your friends, continue to attend as many as you can. It will give you a great opportunity to bounce any struggles you are having with those that know you better than your average acquaintances. Just remember not to share anything too personal with them that could come back to embarrass you or your wife in the future.

YOUR WIFE'S CONTACTS

It was suggested to me not to forget my wife's contacts. Your wife has her own friends, co-workers, and acquaintances. In all of the chaos of getting the word out to the family and your friends, don't forget to make sure her contacts know as well. It's easy to see how she could miss some of them with what is happening.

Again, the reaction will be two-fold. Some of your wife's friends might disappear during this process because of their own emotions toward cancer. But, the majority will rally around her and shower her with love and support. In fact, some of our old neighbors and church friends came out of the woodwork and my wife was able to renew those friendships again.

CANCER BLOG?

One thing you can do is create a contact list of those people that really want to be informed of her progress. I used Facebook to periodically keep our friends up-to-date, but I was given a great suggestion to create a blog that would give a more personal explanation to those people who subscribe. The blog worked great, so you might want to give it a try.

Along this journey, you will make new friends and strengthen relationships with old ones. Those that fade to the background will bounce back in their own time.

Remember not to hold grudges against anyone when they say things that might seem offensive or strange. They may think they are giving you support. You have to make the choice not to be offended at something that was said with good intentions.

You will feel great relief once you get the word out and everyone knows what your family is dealing with.

CHAPTER FIVE

Choosing the Doctors

Once the word gets out, you will be bombarded with doctor recommendations. Everyone's doctor is the best and most qualified . . . as you will quickly learn.

I had experienced doctor recommendations when we were going to have our first child, and everyone was recommending their OB/GYN to my wife. It was nerve-wracking listening to everyone's opinion. As soon as we thought we had it narrowed down, someone would chime up with the news that they knew that doctor and didn't like him or her. It's hard to realize that it's a personality game and your wife will end up choosing the one she feels most comfortable with. In the end, it's her decision.

AT LEAST THREE

The greatest advice my wife and I received was to visit with at least three doctors, and if all the physicians agreed on the same course of action, then choose one of them. If you meet with more than this, you can waste a lot of time and needlessly prolong her decision. Even three can seem daunting, as you will most likely meet with several of their preferred specialists as well.

As I mentioned earlier, my wife's OB/GYN referred us to his wife's cancer surgeon. We were really impressed and my wife could have proceeded with her and been perfectly happy. But we went ahead and set up appointments with two other breast cancer specialists, just to make sure.

NARROWING DOWN YOUR LIST

The nice thing about today's technology is that you can go on to the Internet and get all sorts of information on specialists in your area. My wife and I started with specialists' sites that came highly recommended by people we trusted. We then read patient testimonials of the doctors we were considering. This procedure helped narrow down the choices significantly.

After a few days of fielding emails and phone calls from everyone under the sun, my wife finally settled on two additional doctors and we scheduled the appointments. Once again, we were really impressed.

The recommendations of all three doctors were in harmony, which was a huge relief. My biggest fear was that we might hear something totally different from all three, which would further complicate and delay matters.

Even though I liked all of the physicians, they had different styles. I did not envy my wife's decision. I added a lot of confusion to this process by giving my opinion on all three of them, and it really perplexed her. Do not try to sway her.

Because it was such a personal area that needed to be worked on, I felt she might be more comfortable with a female doctor. But I learned, as we moved along, to wait until she asked for my opinion, and then I could chime in with a supportive answer. Even if you end up not caring for her choice, it is still *her* choice.

BE PATIENT

I think because women tend to have a more personal and emotional relationship with all of their doctors, this process might take a while. If your wife's cancer is caught early, and there is no pressing need for surgery or treatment, give her time. If she is in a more advanced stage, then time is of the essence and you might need to help her decide more quickly.

Once your wife makes her decision, let the other doctors know, and thank them for meeting with you. If your wife feels apprehensive in making these calls, do it for her. It's not fair to the other doctor's offices to keep trying to make appointments if there is no longer any interest. As with any type of business, they will be disappointed in your decision not to use them, but most doctors and medical professionals understand. The doctors my wife did not choose respected her decision and acted professionally. Because of this she was comfortable using one of them on another surgery she needed. They don't want to burn any bridges and neither should you.

OTHER DOCTORS

I mentioned earlier that your doctor would have a team of specialists he or she works with and recommends. For example, it made sense to use the plastic surgeon my wife's breast cancer surgeon worked in tandem with. One of the main reasons my wife felt confident with the plastic surgeon was a book that he had showing the results of the reconstructive surgery. We had a hard time telling the repaired breast from the original one. This information was comforting and helpful, so ask your doctor if a resource like this is available.

If there is a treatment phase before or following surgery, you will most likely meet their preferred medical and radial oncologists. Your wife shouldn't feel like she has to use all of the doctors at one location. My wife used a medical oncologist at one clinic for chemotherapy, and another radial oncologist at a clinic closer to home for her radiation.

It is important that you be there for as many of these visits as you can. You will need to help your wife compare all of the options and recommendations to see how they differ and what suits her best.

ASK QUESTIONS

Once you have heard the recommendations from the different doctors, you need to ask specific questions in relationship to your wife's situation. Ask as many questions as necessary for you to fully understand what is happening. If doctors grow tired of your questioning, you might want to find new ones. They should be very patient and understanding.

I was really impressed with all the doctors that my wife chose to work with. They were all patient with our questions, even though we repeatedly asked the same ones dozens of times. They all took time to explain in detail what she could expect after treatment, the common side effects, and what was coming down the road.

Speaking of down the road, I was amazed at all of the advancements that they shared with us that have happened over the past five years in the various fields of cancer treatment. Thanks to public awareness and increased donations, it's exciting to see where we will be with these treatments in the years to come.

Hopefully, you will regard your doctors as close friends of your family when all is said and done, as they really do have the best interests of your wife at heart.

CHAPTER SIX

Giving Support at Every Turn

After meeting with the doctors, it is on to the surgeries and the treatments. Being able to give your wife the proper support will be paramount in making it as easy on her as possible. In fact, by the time she's through with everything, you will begin to sound and act like a health professional on many fronts.

No matter what your relationship was with your wife prior to her cancer, it has the potential to really improve with this ordeal. To this point you've already survived many of the ups and downs a marriage can throw at you, but the magnitude of this obstacle can seem daunting. I can honestly tell you that our bond became much stronger, and I spoke with dozens of couples that told me the same thing. Now remember, these were couples that stayed together through the *whole* ordeal. If you can stick it out and be with her at every turn, you will find a deeper and more mature level of love you never knew existed.

DON'T TAKE HER FOR GRANTED

I was amazed and ashamed to realize how much I had taken my wife for granted. I was just accustomed to all of the things she would do for me and our family. It's a big reality check when you experience firsthand what a wife and mother does on a daily basis. If you have had to stay home for an extended period of time, you have tasted the hectic schedule that she can keep. When I have done this, I really had a hard time getting anything accomplished that I set out to do. You will most likely experience extended periods of time where you will be keeping her schedule . . . so be prepared.

Unfortunately, an increasing number of husbands, when faced with a life-changing event like this, become overwhelmed and run the other way. Studies show that divorce rates increase due to the stress that cancer causes in a relationship. *I'm here to tell you that you are stronger than this.* Don't let the shock, fear, depression, and stress you both can feel eat away at your relationship. Recognize these negative influences early, and get help if you need it. Reach out to some trusted friends who have navigated through a similar experience that you can confide in or get some counseling. Her cancer will be a battle for you as well, and you will need a lot of support to be able to give her the help she needs. You do not need to feel like you have to handle this by yourself.

IT'S YOUR TURN

I don't know if you are ever prepared for cancer, and when it hits your wife, it can turn your world upside down. Now it's your turn to be the direct and involved caregiver.

When my wife was diagnosed with cancer in her late thirties, I suddenly became aware of how many people had a family member or friend who had cancer in their twenties, thirties, or forties. When you begin to look into cancer studies, you find an increasing number of young men and women diagnosed with cancer. There are many factors discussed in these studies. A lot of them mention environmental pollution, toxic chemicals, preservatives, and processed foods. They all can play a part in breaking down the body's defenses against cancer cells.

Although these studies can be alarming, you will find they are done with the purpose of supporting those who will be impacted by this disease. The research offers hope of eventually eradicating different forms of cancer by changing behavior patterns, improving nutritional habits, and practicing preventative awareness. Even though everyone carries cancer cells in their body, we can make it very difficult for them to bunch together or overrun our systems by applying some of these findings.

ACCEPT SUPPORT

You must be willing to accept support. At first, you may feel overwhelmed with the intrusions in your life and may feel embarrassed by the attention. But the more you allow others to help, the easier it will be to concentrate on your wife.

So what are some of the best ways you can support her?

Gatekeeper

Initial support from family and friends will be a good boost to your wife early on, but once the surgeries and treatments start, too many visits can drain her and become more of a detriment. You will need to be the gatekeeper and support her by keeping visitors at bay when necessary. It's OK to let the phone go to voicemail or not answer the front door when she needs to rest. You can turn the phone ring level down to low and disconnect the doorbell if need be. These can be very nerve-wracking. If you use the social media tips mentioned previously, you can better control the well-wishers and pass along their words of encouragement at more appropriate time.

Scribe

You will need to be the scribe for all doctor's visits. That is why I recommend attending as many as you can. If you cannot be there, have her call you immediately after the appointment and write down everything that was said. Or, have her go with a family member or friend that can take notes. Do not slack off thinking that it's just another doctor's appointment. As mentioned earlier, a lot of the information the doctor will give your wife will be overwhelming to her. Even though you will receive a ton of general information, you will need to write down what the doctors say about your wife's unique situation. Trust me, you will learn great short hand techniques here.

I personally liked keeping a calendar so I could write down what happened and what was said at each visit. As more doctors become involved, they will need to get information from you on when certain treatments were done or tests were performed, so bring the calendar with you to each appointment. This record will also help you in regards to health insurance issues and financial tracking later on.

As scribe, you will play a vital role for others as well. For the rest of your life, if anyone has to care for a loved one with cancer, you will be the one they turn to because of your experience. Your knowledge and experience will be a lifeline for others that need to talk. Your relationship with them will also strengthen.

Children

Most of us fathers work long days and when we get home, we often begrudgingly give our wives a break from the children. But we don't really involve ourselves in the hectic schedule of each child's life . . . we leave that up to her. Now it will be necessary to engage yourself and take the opportunity to build a deeper relationship with each of your children. A great way to support your wife is to support them.

RELATIONSHIP PROFILE

No matter how old your children are, I recommend getting a relationship profile from your wife on each child. She is involved with your children on a different level than you are, and when this relationship gets interrupted, it can really cause stress to both parties. Your wife will feel guilty that she cannot perform her normal routine with them and the children may have a hard time understanding the reasons why.

For younger children at home, the profile your wife creates might include school subjects they're taking and which ones they are struggling in. Your wife is most likely the tutor. She monitors where each kid is academically, makes sure they get to and from school, makes sure they get on their homework after school, and most likely helps all of them with their assignments or projects. I recommend brushing up on your children school subjects. If their curriculum is more advanced than you can handle (and it may well be), the earlier you recognize this, the better. Reach out to the school counselors to get them involved with helping you find appropriate tutors.

You will need to know their favorite activities, snacks, and friends. You'll be amazed at the list your wife can create. She has probably developed a daily schedule and routine with each child. You will need to insert yourself into this schedule or utilize a family member or close friend. You can't just cut this routine off or the children can suffer. If you already know and are familiar with the routine, you will be that much further ahead.

IT'S ABOUT TIME—TO TALK

The best advice I received was to talk with my children. Your children need time to discuss all of those things they would ordinarily share with their mom. They also need to feel that you are really concerned about their day. Listen to them.

This is easier said than done, and may be difficult at first, for all of you. My sisters and I were able to talk to my mom about any subject growing up. Even if it was something that might get us in trouble, our mother was more likely to assess the situation calmly and offer advice . . . whereas our dad had the tendency to overreact. As in most marriages, our father took on the role of disciplinarian, which is why we would hold certain things back from him. I noticed this with my children. I could sense an apprehension from them the first few times my wife had her chemotherapy treatments and couldn't tuck them into bed for a few days afterward. But once they sensed that my interest in listening to them was genuine and I displayed patience with their responses, I noticed our channels of communication were increasing. I found them talking with me more often throughout the day instead of just at bedtime. It was cool that they began to trust me with what they were thinking about and dealing with at school. It reminded me that I had been there myself.

If there is a sporting event, movie, or television program you like to watch to unwind after a long day at work, invest in a DVR or record it so you can see it after they are in bed. If your wife is unable to provide this function and you blow them off to watch television, trust me, they will begin to resent you.

Your wife is also the one most likely to call older children and grandchildren outside of the home to see how things are going. She is the one that plans the family events and parties and the one that sees that school activities are attended. Now it will be your turn to do your best to take on these responsibilities and make yourself available. Make sure they know of your willingness to help out with these functions and follow through whenever you can. Talk is cheap. If you say you will help or show up at functions and fail to follow through, it will be hard to get their trust back.

Parents

When you were married, you promised to have and to hold each other for life. This was the point that you became your own family unit and your parents and her parents were now moved to the "extended family" classification. At my wedding ceremony, the gentlemen officiating said that my wife and I had taken control of our own ship and were beginning to chart our own course. It was at this point he said our parents needed to abandon the ship. You will need to support your wife by knowing when to say when to parental involvement.

As previously mentioned, if my daughter ever goes through something like this, experience has taught me the need to check with her husband to understand in what areas they will need help. Sometimes, parents with good intentions can help too much and cause undue stress to you and your wife. If both sets of parents are always at your house, it won't be long before you get on each other's nerves. Work out a schedule that will be beneficial for everyone.

Make sure that parents have your mobile phone number and work numbers so they can contact you with any questions. Work to make yourself available because if parents have a hard time reaching you, they'll increase their calls to your wife. You might have to explain things over and over again since the stress of the situation can cause parents to forget or misinterpret your conversations. Be patient. Make sure the information you give your parents is not glossed over. Be thorough in your communication. Her parents and your parents need to know exactly what's going on.

The Surgeries

My wife had multiple surgeries, and I was at as many pre-op appointments as possible. Being there gave me the chance to ask the doctor pertinent questions about the procedures and why they were necessary. I recommend you be at as many appointments as possible because your wife will most likely be preoccupied with the surgery itself, but she will have questions of her own. Take time with your wife before the appointments to create a list of questions so she will have her questions answered as well.

Once we arrived at the hospital, I made sure that each doctor who came in to help prep my wife knew her past issues with medications. For instance, she cannot take any narcotic drug without becoming nauseated. When the anesthesiologists came in, I made sure they were aware of this and cautioned them to administer the drugs carefully. If they asked her if she were allergic, she would simply reply "No". But I would have to follow up with, "She may not be allergic, but they can have adverse effects." This is one of the major benefits in having two people present.

If narcotic drugs make your wife very nauseated, have the anesthesiologist try a Total Intravenous Anaesthesia (TIVA), which means that instead of using gas, the narcotics are applied to the IV directly. My wife seemed to handle this better. You can also try a Scopolamine Patch to help with nausea as well. This is a patch that is placed behind the ear that can block the nausea signals to their head. There is a warning, however, make sure they do not touch the patch then touch their eye. If they do, their eyes will be dilated for a day or two.

NO CHILDREN!

Do not make the mistake of bringing children to the hospital unless there is absolutely no one trustworthy to leave them with. The last thing anyone wants is a lot of bored and restless children in the waiting or recovery rooms. I made sure all of my extended family knew exactly when my wife would be having the surgery and arranged well in advance to have them cared for. Do not leave these details until the last minute. There will be plenty of chances for visits once your wife is through with her surgery and over the effects of the anesthesia.

BE A TEAM PLAYER

If you stay at the hospital, try not to whine and complain about your sleeping arrangements, the hospital food, or not having a private bathroom. Buck up and deal with it. You will not get your best night's rest on the La-Z-Boy, love seat, or pullout bed with the bar in the back, but your wife will definitely want you with her. Do not dump this responsibility on your extended family. Even though her parents changed her diaper as a baby, she will feel uncomfortable having them there when she needs to use the restroom or exposes herself in one of those classy hospital gowns.

Once she has rested and her pain is under control, a visit or two from the family will be nice. You will need to get out and stretch your legs or get something to eat. I recommend bringing your own snacks that you can eat inconspicuously throughout your stay. Do not sit down in front of your wife and start pounding a huge meal. One, it could make her sick; and two, it's rude. Hopefully, your hospital will have a few food options for you. If not, most of them are located in a city with plenty of restaurants.

HELP THE NURSES

It is helpful to be aware that the post-surgery monitors and other devices are working properly. After one of my wife's operations, the circulation leg pumps were not plugged back in and I had to get the nurse to hook them up again. Ask precise questions so you know the normal functions and readings of all equipment in her room. Trust me. You will become good at this and will pick up some great nursing skills in the process. Be careful how you talk to the medical staff, however. No one wants to deal with a know-it-all!

No matter how squeamish you are, you will need to be the one to help change the bandages, empty the barf bucket, and service the surgical sites once you're home. Do not pawn this off on your extended family unless absolutely necessary. If at all possible, work from home or work shorter hours until she is able to take care of herself. Any time you can spend together during her recovery will be appreciated. If this is impossible, get someone reliable that you can train to handle her needs and keep an efficient schedule.

Chemotherapy

This is one area where I needed a lot more guidance. How do you effectively support someone who can be dragged through the depths of hell with this kind of treatment? (Sorry to go biblical on you.)

Most of the husbands I reached out to did not go into the details of chemotherapy. The effects can be dreadful and extremely personal. I can see why they held back on the specifics.

You have no idea how your wife will handle each treatment or each type of drug that is administered. Each one comes with its own set of side effects. Be prepared to support her in a number of related areas.

DRUG TYPES

Become knowledgeable as to what type of drug will be administered and its side effects. The oncologist will tell you that she might experience a few side effects or even all of them. Not that you should be a fatalist, but it is better to be pleasantly surprised if they are minimal than utterly disappointed if the majority of them rear their ugly heads.

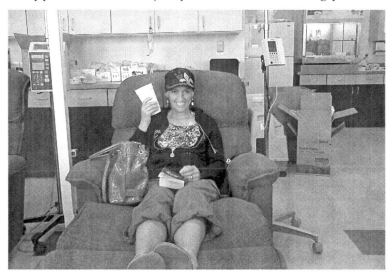

Cindy putting on her happy face for one of her chemotherapy appointments . . . attitude is everything!

You will quickly learn what is normal and what is not. Be prepared for anything.

My wife had three different chemo drugs. All of them were required to rid her of any hidden cancer cells and worked on different areas of her body. They also killed her body's immune system for fighting infection and viruses.

One drug called Epirubicin was nicknamed the "Red Devil." If it touched your skin it would eat it away like an acid. But when slowly carried into the blood stream through injection, it had no adverse effect on the arteries. My wife could actually feel the medicine go into her body. The other two were called Cytoxan and Taxotere.

I V ' S

You will most likely have to take her to get IV fluids if she cannot stomach food for a few days. If you can, take multiple days off work or work from home following each treatment. Do not assume that a few sips of water or other liquids is enough to stave off dehydration. Follow the recommendations given by your oncologist. You will need to monitor this. If it is common that she requires IV appointments soon after her first couple of treatments, make sure they are scheduled well in advance of her remaining treatments so the oncology facility is ready to accomodate you.

The majority of cancer patients will also need multiple shots of a drug called Neupogen administered daily for up to two weeks after each treatment. This helps their body reproduce the white blood cells needed to fight illness.

FOOD HUNTER

A good thing you can do is encourage her to try a variety of liquids and foods to see which ones she can tolerate. Similar to when a woman is pregnant, if she has a craving for anything . . . go get it! You will become Meals on Wheels. Try to avoid spicy, sweet, fatty, or salty foods. Bland is a good rule of thumb, especially right after a treatment.

My wife seemed to tolerate smoothies, so the local smoothie joint became a frequent stop for me. It's the same experience as teaching your children to eat. You just keep trying until they find something they like. My wife and I were both ecstatic when that would happen!

You wouldn't think there would be any drug out there that would keep liquids from being refreshing. I was wrong. Her drugs caused a mouth infection called Thrush. Everything she drank had a horrible metallic taste. She described the liquid texture like trying to swallow cotton balls. About the only thing she could tolerate was flat ginger ale. Some people do better with a liquid diet a day before and a day after treatment to avoid upsetting the stomach too much.

Be patient and don't give up. Hopefully, you will receive some good suggestions from others on what worked for them. I received great information at her chemo appointments from the nurses and fellow patients. Write these down and note those that show up multiple times, and your chances for success will increase.

Do not eat at your favorite restaurants during treatments. If you do, they will remind her of the chemo and it may be a while before she can eat there again. I've talked with many couples that cannot even drive by their favorite places anymore. If she is craving her favorite entrée get it "to go" and bring it home so there will be less of a connection.

GERM EXTERMINATOR

Because the immune system is compromised during treatments, you have to be aware of infections and viruses. This includes keeping anyone away who is sick, making sure pets are not crawling all over her, using anti-bacterial wipes constantly, and letting family and friends know about each appointment so they won't drop by unexpectedly.

My wife's immune system was at its lowest level about six or seven days after a treatment, so we had very little outside contact with anyone for a few days until the Neupogen shots increased her white blood cell count. Be ready at a second's notice for any sign of illness or fever as she will not be able to fight it without going to the ER for antibiotics. Call the doctor immediately if a fever of 100.5 degrees develops or if she has chills.

HAIR LOSS

Within two weeks of the first chemo treatment, my wife's hair began falling out. Even though you are warned this may happen it is still shocking. My wife decided to be proactive and shave her hair off before it fell out so it would be less of a mess.

My wife always had thick, long hair, so we were worried about how the children would react to a bald mom. Other husbands that I knew had shaved their heads as a sign of solidarity between them and their wives, so I decided to do the same. I had never shaved my head before, but it was the least I could do.

With the help of my wife's friend, we both shaved our heads at the same time. I went first to lessen the shock for our children and to take some of the focus off my wife. By the time it was her turn, the children were excited to help cut her hair. Before long, our oldest son, nephews, brothers-in-law, and even some neighbors shaved their heads to show support.

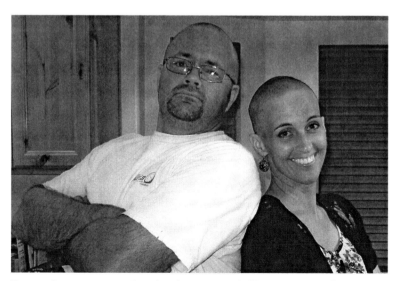

If my wife was going to lose her hair so was I. Shaving our heads together.

NAUSEA

For at least seven to ten days after each of her eight treatments, it was all up to me. She spent most of those days in our bedroom or bathroom feeling horribly nauseated. She tried many different drugs for nausea, but nothing worked well.

Too much light made her nauseated. Smells in the house made her nauseated. The only way I could support her was by letting her stay where she was and just manage through it. I wanted to help relieve the pain and discomfort, but I couldn't. It was sobering.

Chemo is when you really earn your "stripes."

It will seem like a long process, and test you and your wife on many levels. She will not feel well and you might need to be her emotional punching bag for a while, but better you than anyone else. Learn to cope with the ups and downs as best you can.

Radiation Therapy

The advancement in radiation treatment has given people options. Make sure you are aware of which ones are available and get feedback on the pros and cons from as many people as possible. Once the radial oncologist and your wife decide what type of laser treatment to use, make sure you understand the markings and what preparations need to be made before your wife's visit. They will most likely need to tattoo the area with small markings to make sure the laser beams hit the targeted area. Familiarize yourself with that area and help your wife monitor any abnormalities.

Supporting your wife through radiation can range in complexity depending on the area that needs to be treated. I recommend going to the first couple of treatments to see how they affect her and also to make sure your wife is comfortable getting to and from the treatments safely. I also recommend attending the last round of treatments, as the treatment area will be tender and painful by this time.

Compared to chemo, my wife's radiation treatments and side effects were less severe. There was some mild fatigue and sunburn redness around the radiated area. Other than the forty-five minute daily appointment she had for a few weeks, she was able to keep a normal routine.

BAGGY CLOTHES

Make sure your wife has some loose fitting clothing. The radiated site can become irritated and it is better for her to wear things that are not too tight. Loose blouses and sweaters were my wife's favorites. Those who experienced other cancers recommended drawstring shorts and pajama bottoms.

Medications

This is one area you will have to monitor like a hawk. My wife was not accustomed to taking a lot of medication, so for her to remember to take some pills four times a day and others two times a day was challenging. At one point she was taking Zofran for nausea, Bactrim as an antibiotic, and Loritab for pain. Her doctors also instructed her to take nutritional supplements like iron, if her blood count was low in certain areas. Some pills would have to be taken with food, while others worked better between meals. I got used to setting an alarm clock or timer on our stove to help remind her until she got into the habit of taking them as prescribed.

I recommend purchasing a slotted pill case that has compartments for each day of the week. They are available at any pharmacy drugstore. These cases help monitor that she is taking the proper amount.

DATE NIGHTS

When your wife feels well enough, a regularly scheduled date night is one of the best ways to give her a boost. If you have maintained a good routine throughout your marriage, do not stop now even though your schedule will get more hectic. If you have let this aspect of your relationship slide, then now is the time to revive it. You will both need the one-on-one time together more than ever.

Communication is King

The days of staying up until the wee hours talking about "whatever" may seem like forever ago and we can hit phases in our marriage where we get so busy with other things that we forget how to truly communicate. She may not be able to open up to you at home with all of the distractions. Getting her away so you can be alone will help. Take advantage of every opportunity that presents itself.

Make sure you go to places that permit close communication. Going to movies, loud restaurants, or sporting events do not give you that opportunity. Getting some ice cream and going to a park are better options.

It was recommended to me to let her pick the topics of conversation. At first, all I wanted to talk about was her cancer, not realizing that she might want to talk about something else. You will have plenty of opportunities to discuss that elsewhere. I learned to keep subjects light and incorporated as much humor as I could. It was difficult at first, but together we decided to leave the reality of the disease alone for a while.

These moments will also be a great time to see if there are other areas that concern her and require your assistance.

CHAPTER SEVEN

Household Chores

Laundry and Shopping and Cooking — Oh My!

Other responsibilities your wife might need assistance with will most likely include many household chores, which may be totally foreign to you. You might handle the garbage, mow the lawn, repair household items, maintain the cars, or whip up some soup once in a while . . . but she most likely handles most of the cooking, dishes, laundry, shopping, ironing, sewing, vacuuming, dusting, pets, planting, etc. Do you see where I'm going with this? Your wife's day can involve so much more than you realize.

I feel my wife said it best in a poem she wrote years ago.

Uniforms a Mother Wears

The uniforms a mother wears changes frequently,

It all depends on what goes on within her family.

Morning comes, she's Boot Camp Sergeant waking up her crew.

She blows the whistle, shakes the bed . . . that camouflage is new.

Rakes, gloves, and shovels, a T-shirt and faded jeans,

There goes the gardener, to plant a row of beans.

Sometimes she's a nurse, to mend the scratch or bruise.

Other times she's cheerleader, to support you, win or lose.

The uniform a mother wears changes with every hour.

What will that mother soon become when she steps out of the shower?

She's zipping up her jumpsuit to go and fix a flat.

Bicycle repairman! Can you imagine that?

Tennis shoes and flip-flops, boots of every type.

Is that mom a janitor, from all the floors she wipes?

Here she is the hairdresser, to help the kids look right.

Now she comes in striped shirt to referee the fight.

The uniform a mother wears changes frequently.

Running errands, making stops . . . like having her own taxi.

At dinnertime, the apron's on and she becomes the cook.

At bedtime she's librarian, who reads the kids a book.

As she tucks in all the children, I believe she's wearing wings,

For she sounds just like an angel, as she softly sings.

What uniform does she like best? I think it all depends

On what job is most important among family and friends.

The majority of husbands I know are the main breadwinners of their family and help with chores as best they can, but their wives still have more responsibility running the home.

DOMESTIC TORCH

If you were living the dream of coming home from work with a warm, cooked meal on the table, your wife refreshed and all dressed up to greet you, the children well-behaved and eager to show you their latest honorary science projects, then get ready because things are about to change. The domestic torch is about to be passed on to you!

Think about what we have discussed so far.

After most surgeries, your wife will need time to recuperate and will be instructed not to lift much of anything. She will be told to ease back into general household duties. I can't count how many doctors and nurses told us that my wife could not lift anything heavier than a gallon of milk for two to three weeks after every surgery. Almost everything weighs more than a gallon of milk!

During chemotherapy, your wife will not have the energy to do the most basic chores for days or even weeks. Getting up from the bed to the bathroom will require all the strength she has. The smells of everything around the house will most likely set her off, which will really limit her ability to monitor the shape of things.

Even radiation can throw your wife's days out of rhythm because her treatments will most likely be during the middle of the day and fatigue can set in soon after.

The fact I'm trying to stress is that you will be responsible for creating new household routines for yourself and your children, while your wife deals with getting well. You will have to do all of this and still maintain your employment demands. Don't wait until the torch is given to you. Get some training from your wife on how to man the household battle stations.

As soon as your wife is diagnosed, and you know what treatments she will need, sit down and make a list of the things she does every day and how often. Use another calendar to track the days she does certain chores. (Can you tell I'm a big proponent of calendars?)

THE DREADED CHORES

I have yet to meet a man that likes to do the following, so I wanted to mention these as they might be ones you haven't had to tackle for a while.

Laundry

You'll be surprised at how quickly the laundry can stack up after only a few days. My wife, for short stretches during her treatments, did not have the energy to sort the laundry, haul it to the washer, then the dryer, iron it, and put it away. Your wife will need to train you on *her* way of doing it, because if it is done wrong, she might insist on doing it herself. My wife felt guilty, at first, that I had to do one of her main duties and was struggling to get the hang of it. But, as long as you have the right attitude in taking it over, she will feel better about allowing you to.

Here are some laundry tips:

- Don't try to cheat and wash everything in cold water, thinking colors won't bleed. This might have worked for you in college, but if she sees articles of different colors going in at the same time, no matter how cold you say the water is, your plan will be shot down.
- If she does allow you to mix colors, be wary of new clothes, as they need to be washed a few times with similar colors before you can combine them and cut corners.
- Make sure whites are washed by themselves, no matter what, as sometimes cold water is not cold enough and other colors will bleed. Better safe than sorry in this situation.
- If you have items in the dryer that will wrinkle, stay within buzzer distance and as soon as you hear it, go hang up the clothes so you do not have to iron them. You can always put them back in the dryer with a wetted washcloth if you forget, but anything is better than ironing. Save yourself some burns.
- Teach your children to do the sniff test with their clothes and if it doesn't stink, have them wear it again.

I know that sounds harsh. Maybe it's the difference
between husbands and wives, but I was surprised
how quickly my children would go through wardrobe
changes every day. This taught them that having their
laundry done for them is a privilege and not a right.

- Make sure not to wash anything that says, "Dry Clean
  Only". Double-check your wife's or daughter's clothing because they seem to have more of these items
  than males do. Leave hand washing to Grandma!

Clothes Shopping

If your children need clothes, wait until your wife is well
enough to go with them or send them with a family member or friend that likes to shop. They will know what they
are doing. Do not try to figure out what is cool for your
children . . . especially your daughters. Hopefully, you or
your wife will have someone you trust to help out with the
clothes shopping.

If you are going to tackle clothes shopping, make sure
you have their sizes written down on those profiles I mentioned earlier and make a list of things they need. I made the
mistake of going without a list. I came back with a bunch
of items on sale that no one would wear, so I wasted a lot
of time with returns. Remember, a sale is worthless if they
don't need it or won't wear it! Clothes shopping takes planning, so the more help you get the better.

Cooking

When your wife goes through her nausea phases of treatment, you will need to be the one that plans and cooks the meals. You will either be doing this for your family or yourself. Most husbands have a few dinners we can throw together, but we haven't had to do it consistently for an extended period of time. If you end up making the same menu over and over again, you and your children will get burned out. Some of us might be able to live off ramen noodles, like we did in college, but your children won't.

On the flip side, if you give up cooking and try the fast food route every night, it will get old. You need to maintain a variety of home-cooked meals (with the occasional trip to McDonalds to make the children happy) to be sure you are eating the way you should.

If your wife is having treatments during the summer or days when your children are out of school, you need to become adept at preparing a wide variety of meals that cover breakfast, lunch, and dinner. This will be stressful for you at first, but you will get the hang of it with proper planning.

Sit down and lay out a few weeks' worth of meals with your wife and a list of all necessary staples. If you do this, you can use this list again and again without the children noticing the same meal patterns. They won't mind tacos every three weeks but they will mind them every Wednesday. Make sure to space time between ethnic foods as well. You might be able to handle Italian every night, but your kids will get pasta overload. If you rotate potatoes, rice, and pasta you will have enough varieties of some pretty cheap staples.

Grocery Shopping

Most husbands are familiar with the magazine section, pharmacy, and automotive areas of a grocery store, but we get lost if we have to find gravy mix or taco seasoning. Make sure you get to know your local supermarket. Spend a little time and see how it is laid out. Learn to get the non-perishable items first, then the refrigerated and frozen items last. It's sad to get home with two pounds of warm meat you don't dare eat.

When shopping, make sure you bring a shopping list. Do not try to do it by memory. Trust me . . . you will not remember everything.

Resist the urge to buy chips, soft drinks, and doughnuts. You're trying to cultivate good nutrition and when your wife is ready to eat, she will need healthy choices.

HIGH FIBER & ANTIOXIDANT DIET

A diet high in fiber and antioxidants is recommended. These foods include anything with a high content of bran, brown or wild rice, whole wheat bread, pasta, sweet potatoes, broccoli, carrots, corn, asparagus, spinach, apricots, strawberries, apples, blueberries, cantaloupe, and oranges.

Make sure you familiarize yourself with some of the nutritional studies that have been done for a full list of these foods. You might be surprised how much you and your family will learn to like them—with a little encouragement. (Although a small bag of Cheetos won't hurt once in a while!)

IT'S ALL IN THE ATTITUDE

As with most things in life, the right attitude can make all the difference. If you are positive and learn to embrace these additional "opportunities," you will be surprised at what you can accomplish. The knowledge of how to tackle these domestic duties can only help you move forward.

> *Nothing can stop the man with the right mental attitude from achieving his goal; nothing on earth can help the man with the wrong mental attitude.* —*Thomas Jefferson*

CHAPTER EIGHT

The Costs

In many marriages, one spouse is the saver or penny pincher and the other spouse is the spender. I admit that I was the spender and my wife the saver. After many years, I began to see the reasoning for saving money for a rainy day, and I have eventually come over to her side . . . more often than not.

If both spouses are savers, then kudos to you. You probably feel more prepared for what life throws your way. If you both spend every penny you make, you most likely live paycheck to paycheck and live with financial stress. No matter which end of the spectrum you're on, when cancer comes along, it can throw a fifty-pound wrench into the financial engine of your marriage.

In most cases, you do not budget for a catastrophic medical issue like cancer. Unless someone who has been through this shares their financial details, you will have no idea of the costs involved. Hopefully, there will be some kind of financial support that can relieve some or most of the burden.

MEDICAL/HEALTH INSURANCE

I used to complain all the time about having to pay for medical insurance at work. It seemed like every year premiums would increase, programs paid for by my employer would be dropped, and coverage areas and in-network choices would shrink. Bottom line . . . I felt like insurance was a huge waste of money.

The few times my family used our benefits didn't seem to outweigh the amount deducted from my check each pay period. Not to mention, the money I was putting into my company's Health Savings Account (HSA) program.

Well, I don't complain anymore.

I had no idea what the costs of cancer would be. Looking at all of the medical bills and insurance statements over an 18-month period put the overall cost in the hundreds of thousands range . . . and we're still not through! After comparing my insurance plan's out-of-pocket maximum with the overall costs, my costs were mere pocket change.

If your wife was just diagnosed, and you have time to do it before your next renewal period, go with the lower deductible-higher cost plan your company might offer. Even though you will have more money taken out of your check, the maximum out-of-pocket amount will be easier to come up with.

Some other tips I have learned along the way include:

- Stay in-network: We did not even visit with any doctors who were out-of-network because we were afraid we would like them more than those on our plan. Do not underestimate the discounts your insurance company gets when working with in-network doctors and hospitals. Be sure to check your company's insurance website for these providers before making any appointments.

- Lump sum payments: Once your insurance has paid for a service and you receive your portion of the bill, call the billing department and ask if they offer a paid-in-full discount. Hopefully, you will have some money saved and be able to pay them in one lump sum, as it will usually save you between ten to forty percent.

- Be organized: Keep every claim notice from your insurance company and the corresponding bill. Sometimes the same service will be billed twice under another claim number. You only need to pay for a service once. *Watch for duplicate claims!* Get to know your insurance company's website. Claims for each member of your family will be listed for any specified period and organized by date. Make a printout, and compare it with the notices and bills to be sure everything is accurate. You may have to call the billing departments and your insurance company multiple times to get these fixed. Better to jump on them early than try to deal with them years later when things are more difficult to research.

- Your portion: If a billing department statement shows a smaller payment amount than your insurance notice does, do not blow this difference off thinking you got away with something. This discrepancy could go to a collection agency or end up hurting your credit if not paid. Let the billing department know how much your insurance company says you owe so they can verify the correct amount. If billed later, you will miss out on the savings of the lump sum discount mentioned above.

- Out-of-pocket max: Once you have met the out-of-pocket max deductible, 100% of services should be covered by your insurance company. Know exactly when you reach this point so you can avoid double payments because hospital or clinic refunds can take several weeks. If there is some other medical need in your family, you might as well take care of it now that the deductible is met. For example, if your child needs to get his or her tonsils out or you have put off that ingrown wart on your foot, go for it.

The bottom line is that your insurance company should be sensitive and understanding to what you are going through. If you have problems with your insurance company, get your HR department from work involved.

I have nothing but good things to say about my insurance company and how everything was handled by all parties. The majority of communications I received from them were detailed and easy to understand. On occasion, we would receive a decline of coverage notice, but it had to deal with the information the hospital was providing and I would have to make a quick call to verify the information needed was sent. These instances were limited and well worth my inquiries to make sure everyone was on the same page.

If you're between jobs, it can be a scary time to have major medical bills or impending medical events. I remember before the birth of my second child, I was laid off and had to pick up COBRA insurance. Although it was a great safety net, I was relieved to start with another company before the delivery, as the deductible would have wiped out our savings.

NO HEALTH INSURANCE?

If you don't have health insurance, you are not alone. There are millions of people who are in the same boat. Contact your local health department regarding information about doctors, hospitals (public and non-profit), and facilities that will treat your wife. Hill-Burton Act hospitals are an example of hospitals that are required to treat cancer patients who can't afford the payments at a regular hospital. Most of these hospitals have social workers that will help you set up a payment plan that will work within your budget.

With or without insurance, there are ways you can raise funds to help pay for deductibles and medical costs. Don't feel like there are no options. Reach out to family, friends, clergy, and cancer survivor groups in your area. In doing so, you will be surprised at the financial support you can receive.

Some of this help can come in the form of meals. Take the money you would've spent on groceries and put it in a savings account earmarked for medical bills. Do the same with any cash donations, as well as money that can come from fundraisers or bake sales.

Learn to budget better. It was recommended that I make a list of all our expenditures and separate what was needed and what was frivolous. By avoiding unnecessary spending, you can free up more funds. Once these income streams are realized, make sure you earmark them properly. Do not be tempted to tap into these funds for other purposes. They are for your wife, not you. Do not use these funds to fix up the house or make other purchases. If people see a need to help in a certain area and want to make the purchase to help, then by all means accept it. Our washing machine went out while we were right in the middle of my wife's chemo treatments and my in-laws stepped in and bought us a new one. It was one of the many financial blessings we received.

IT SHOULD BE YOUR WORRY

The finances need to be your worry and not your wife's. Leave her out of the financial aspect as much as possible.

This is where you need to do your best to have conversations about these matters in private. I tried not to complain about the difficulties I was having in getting things paid. There will be issues between your insurance company and the services rendered that will be a headache working through. But don't make your stress her stress.

Learn to stave off the feelings of financial depression. Early on, I felt it creeping up on me when I would have to write checks out of our savings account that had been earmarked for projects around our home or our family vacation. You'll come to realize what is really important in life, and this will change your view on money.

If you find you're not able to deal with the money stress, take advantage of financial counseling that can be offered through your insurance company or the hospitals where your wife had her surgeries and treatments. It can be a great help to discuss these worries and gather additional ideas.

In worst-case scenarios, these costs can end up driving some into medical bankruptcy, but these counselors will try to help you avoid such a drastic step. It's in everybody's best interest to work together.

CHAPTER NINE

Other Common Emotions

*I've always thought of myself as a levelheaded person . . .
not too high, not too low. Yes, I was susceptible to a little
road rage now and again. Occasionally, I'd shed some tears
at happy or sad moments, but I always felt in control of my
emotions. Until this!*

Cancer changed my emotions when my wife was diagnosed. I noticed I was more emotional and these feelings would come over me without warning. You might notice this as well. You'll never know when or where these feelings will manifest themselves, but you are about to join your wife on a roller coaster of emotional extremes.

As discussed earlier, shock and fear seemed to be the earliest emotions that presented themselves to me, but a few other reactions appeared later on.

DEPRESSION

Depression snuck up on me quite often in different forms. I found myself not caring about many things. Negative thoughts of, "Why did this happen to 'her' and to 'us'?" continually crept into the forefront of my mind, and beat on me constantly. I didn't feel like getting outside and doing many of the things I liked to do.

The only way I could pull out of these moments was to immerse myself in each phase of her cancer treatment. Once I realized their necessity, the process helped me keep my mind focused, and I was less likely to slip into negative thought patterns. It became easier to cope with.

The more you study about cancer and realize how prevalent this disease is, the more you understand that most people will have to deal with it at some point. I don't want to say that misery loves company, but the isolation you first feel can be quelled by this realization. You will gain a new perspective on the medical field and advancements in technology that will help you fight this feeling. You really do have millions of others in your corner.

You begin to think less of "why" it happened and more on "what" can be done about it.

You're not alone.

ANXIETY

The course of your wife's treatment can take anywhere from six to eighteen months—or longer—depending on her type of cancer. Not knowing how she'll respond to procedures, drugs, surgeries, etc., can create a lot of anxiety.

In our technological age, we're used to getting our information quickly and with little effort. With medical websites, we can ask questions and get information with a few strokes on our keyboards. In other words, we have become incredibly impatient.

You must have patience when it comes to medical issues that deal with cancer. The sooner you come to this realization the less anxious you will feel.

Results from tests, screenings, treatments, and other procedures can take weeks. Fight the urge to get impatient with medical personnel, as they are not purposely dragging their feet. They are as concerned with finding out the results as quickly as you are, so they know what they are dealing with and what the appropriate treatment options will be. Most hospitals have cancer boards where multiple doctors will discuss your wife's case in detail and try to compare it to other cases they have treated that are similar. There are so many different variables that go into a proper course of treatment, but know that their recommendations come from many years of experience.

I learned early on, I would rather have them check, and recheck, and debate my wife's results than rush to a conclusion and start a treatment strategy that wasn't appropriate.

It is better they get the correct determinations the first time, rather than force a decision based on your own impatience. Depending on the stage and type of cancer, a best-case procedural protocol can then be established.

Keep calm. Help them help your wife by not forcing the process.

ANGER AND RESENTMENT

My wife is one of the healthiest people I have ever met. She exercises regularly; watches what she eats; refrains from drinking alcohol, caffeine, or soft drinks; and does not smoke. It took me years to get her to eat red meat and she only does that occasionally. Other than a torn ACL from playing indoor soccer, she had never had any major health problems.

Then this happened to her and I kept asking, "Why her? How could someone so healthy get a disease like cancer?" It was these thoughts that lead to anger and resentment.

I would look around at the people who were in the doctor's office and clinics and my wife did not belong there. If she were a life-long smoker, worked with cancer-causing chemicals, or was subjected to chemicals in a war, I would have had an easier time understanding.

Indeed, what you eat, things you take into your body, and other lifestyle choices can increase the chances of cancer; but, family genetics and history can play just as large a part in getting cancer or other diseases. For example, some marathon runners have higher cholesterol levels than couch potatoes.

Every doctor we met with pointed out the indiscriminate nature of cancer. It targets whom it targets. Some people can chain-smoke into their nineties without it ever surfacing, while a new baby can be born with it. It's a disease that is out of our control most of the time. After many appointments, I finally realized this and let go of the anger and resentment.

This made it easier for me to have compassion for those that are fighting the disease, and to stop judging how or why they got it.

PARANOIA

Paranoia was one of the strangest emotions for me to get a handle on.

It hit me hardest when I would have to pay a bill. I began to wonder if the doctors were making things up to get more business. Cancer treatments are not cheap, and as the medical claims began to roll in, I started questioning every service. I couldn't help but wonder if they were telling us she needed them so they could make more money. Remember, you're talking about hundreds of thousands of dollars.

I kept envisioning myself involved in some sort of medical conspiracy like in Erin Brockovich.

"Maybe the government is involved and is protecting its medical business interests like it protects its oil interests."

"Maybe my wife's x-rays from her knee injury were the cause of this. The hospitals know it and are not telling anyone."

"Maybe other, less costly treatments half way around the world are more effective and they're not telling us."

Etc., etc., etc. . . . .

STOP IT!

Nobody is out to get you. Once you learn about the medical advancements that are being made in detection and treatment, you will realize the medical field is trying to eradicate cancer . . . not foster it. The government is actively helping to fund cancer research, not deter it.

Occasionally, you will read about a doctor that misdi-agnoses patients to get more business, but those cases are so rare. With all of the medical malpractice suits being brought before the courts you can see why they want to be as thorough as possible.

I watch too many movies and read too many books about conspiracy theories . . . can you tell? You might want to avoid these forms of media if you're prone to entertain these types of thoughts.

JEALOUSY

What a selfish emotion jealousy is, especially during a time like this. But it can happen more often than you think.

After my wife was diagnosed, I was willing to discuss her progress with everyone who showed interest and it was comforting to know so many cared. But the longer it went on, the more I realized no one asked about me anymore. I began to feel like I was invisible. When we were together and saw people we knew, I was bypassed completely. Even my children seemed to ignore me more often. I felt like I was doing so much and no one was noticing.

You have to understand no one is doing this on purpose. People that really care about you will naturally be worried about the biggest part of your life, which should be your wife. What concern they show for her should let you know they care for you.

Your wife needs this attention now more than ever. How would she feel if everyone acted disinterested or as though everything were normal? I cringe to even fathom the thought. Hearing from you who asked about her that day and relaying their words of encouragement will lift her spirits and, in turn, lift yours.

The gifts, the flowers, the letters, and the cards not only help her, but they can also help you sweep away these envious feelings that may crop up from time to time.

As these and other emotions surface, never lose sense of your responsibility as her husband. Learn to deal with any negative emotion you feel before it consumes you.

If by nature you're prone to depression and negative emotions, *get help now*. Reach out to others, read self-help books, and/or get counseling. You will need to learn skills to be able to control yourself and handle the added responsibility.

> *Painful as it may be, a significant emotional event can be the catalyst for choosing a direction that serves us —and those around us —more effectively. Look for the learning.*
> —Louisa May Alcott

CHAPTER TEN

Romance

Romance and Cancer Do Not Mix!

I thought I would get this out of the way right now.

Physical attraction and sex are important for the male species. It might sound shallow, but it's true. Women can usually list multiple qualities they want in a man, and romantic aspects will be ranked all over the place in terms of importance. But for men, they're almost always at the top.

There are romantic peaks and valleys in every relationship; and, hopefully, your peaks have been greater than the valleys up to this point. For instance, in my marriage we experienced peaks when we were trying to have children, then we would hit a valley during her pregnancy.

WHY DOES IT CHANGE?

All you need to do is read the studies and reports in your cancer materials to confirm that you are about to enter an extraordinarily long valley. Chemo treatments, due to the drugs, can lower her sexual desire. Surgeries can make sex difficult and painful. Radiation can cause irritation and soreness.

The negative emotions you can experience as you deal with different phases of her cancer might preoccupy your thoughts, which in turn, can affect your desire. Days can quickly turn into weeks, weeks into months. Before you realize it, you haven't even attempted to strike up any romance. Not to mention that when you do, you will most likely be met with rejection—which doesn't help.

Physical Changes

Some reasons this happens may be due to the physical changes from surgeries and chemotherapy.

Helping my wife take care of her surgical sites from her mastectomies hit both of us hard. The difficulty for her was the private nature of the area involved. For me it was seeing an attractive part of her body disfigured. Instead of stimulating romantic desire, that part of her body became an enemy that could've taken her from me. It affected me more than I thought it would.

With most chemotherapy drugs, your wife will not only lose the hair on her head, but she will most likely lose it everywhere. Seeing your wife in this state might be traumatic for you, as well as for her. She almost becomes unrecognizable. You will get used to it, but it will take some time.

Don't be the one to point out all of these changes. She will notice them and you will only make her feel more self-conscious. Do not forget that she is still the same dynamic and beautiful person you married. How you treat her during this ordeal will tell her a lot about you. Step up to the plate and show her the love she deserves.

Emotional Romance

Use this time to connect emotionally. Emotional bonding will allow the physical bonding to simmer on the back burner for a while. The balance of the two will return eventually, but why not nurture this aspect of your relationship for now.

Because of all of the time spent together going through this process, you will be reminded of the reasons you fell in love. You will be able to reconnect with the things you have in common. You will be able to discuss religious views you share and how they can help you get through this. You will get practice in handling her emotional extremes and learn how to deal with your own. Your circle of emotional support connections will grow with the doctors and other people you meet. Fellow survivors and their families will become some of your best friends.

You will start to recognize positive emotional changes in yourself that will come from this experience. Because of these changes, you will begin to see your wife in a new light. Older feelings will resurface and new ones will be forged.

The attentiveness you show her and the acceptance you demonstrate will have lasting dividends with your relationship going forward.

Love is composed of a single soul inhabiting two bodies.
—*Aristotle*

CHAPTER ELEVEN

Your Health

Unfortunately, you may know of someone that has gone off the deep end when faced with a crisis such as this and they start abusing alcohol or drugs to mask or escape the situation. Your own experience might not be this extreme, but it's important to note that detrimental habits can form.

I found comfort in a lot of habits that were not good for me. For example, it was tough to find time or have the energy to exercise. It was easier to watch television or a movie once I got everything settled.

Since I was the main grocery shopper for an extended period of time, I found myself buying and consuming a lot of "comfort foods" with no nutritional value.

Mentally and physically, I neglected myself for a good portion of the first year that my wife was going through this. It was difficult to worry about myself when I was so worried about her and the children. There were things that I liked keeping up with like sports, politics, news, and current events, stuff that really didn't seem to matter as much.

It wasn't until I realized that my clothes were tighter, my focus was shorter, and my stamina was lower that I needed to get back to the basics of taking care of myself.

EATING RIGHT

Because your wife's appetite changes and fluctuates, you can really get into some bad habits of eating whatever and whenever she eats. Your wife's eating habits will be very sporadic. She will most likely not feel like eating at dinnertime, but at many different times during the day. If she craves something, you might find yourself eating right alongside her, without even thinking about it or without being hungry.

It seemed like I ate so much when I was home from work that I was never hungry. Between all of the meals provided by family and friends, as well as the goodies that came flooding in, there was never a want for food.

When we didn't have meals delivered, I had a bad habit of just stopping on the way home from work and getting burgers or pizza to feed the family because it was quick and easy.

As I mentioned earlier, you really need to come up with a meal plan and brush up on your food pyramid knowledge from grade school.

Plan healthy dishes that will keep your strength up and give your immune system the boost it needs. You will receive an incredible amount of nutritional advice in all of her literature, so use it on yourself as well.

EXERCISE

Now is the time to make a change for the better.

You have probably noticed that there are many studies that have shown how exercise can reduce certain types of cancer. So, in an effort to make a positive lifestyle change, why not get started now and get a basic routine going? As soon as your wife is able, get her involved as well.

So what can you do?

Try to find the time to get out and do some good walking, biking, swimming, or running. Outside is a better option than indoors, as the fresh air will help clear your mind and give you time to make assessments. The walls will begin to close in on you if you do not allow yourself time to escape the house for a while. Cardio will also help keep your immune system up, help cut down on depression, and give you increased energy.

Cancer can be a wake-up call to the whole family to get in better shape, so set the example. You might be pleasantly surprised if your children join in as well.

SPIRITUALITY

For a lot of people, spirituality and a belief in God has been a driving force in their lives. It gives them a blueprint on how to live and how to treat others. They understand and accept that there is a higher purpose than just this mortal existence.

If you fall into this category, do not neglect it. Your life will become hectic, but do not put this aspect of your life aside. You will need to have the help of those that share your beliefs. You might also want to reach out to your ecclesiastical leaders for some counsel and support. Just make sure you keep your church attendance and study habits as normal as possible.

Many times I've heard people blame God during stressful times like these and shy away from spirituality. But, if you hold true to your core beliefs, you will be amazed at the well of strength you will receive. Instead of this ordeal driving you from your values, allow it to steer you back to the basics and help you come to terms with this life situation.

HOBBIES & ACTIVITIES

You need to keep doing activities or hobbies that you enjoy—within reason.

I say "within reason" as you really need to be available to your wife. If you're a hunter that takes off for a few weeks while she is recovering or going through treatment, she will not be happy. If your activities or hobbies take you away from home for extended periods of time, it would be wise to alter or develop new ones that can keep you closer.

As an avid golfer, I tried to get out as often as I could just to focus on something other than the reality of the situation.

It really did recharge my batteries. Even though my wife did not golf, she still felt it was important for me to get out once in a while. I really appreciated her support. Many of the men I spoke with said that this was an essential part of keeping themselves together.

It is also important to do activities that can include your children. It gives you a chance to further bond with them and give your wife some uninterrupted time. When she feels up to it, encourage her to do some activities that are new to all of you. For instance my wife went horseback riding to get out and try something different. Who says you can't build some positive memories while working through all of the negative ones?

You need to be operating on all cylinders—emotionally, spiritually, and physically—in order to effectively assist her. Do not let pride get in the way.

Stay strong in all three areas and you will be able to deal with anything thrown your way.

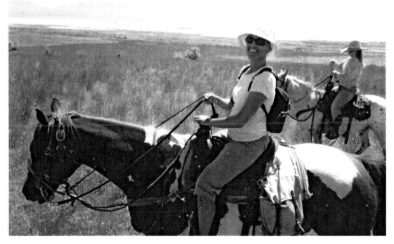

Who says you cannot try new things while getting treatments. Cindy doing some horseback riding.

CHAPTER TWELVE

Your Job

Do not think that in a job-related scenario you are the only one affected by what's going on in your life. For many of us, the people we work with can become a second family. What affects the "one" can affect the "many."

WHO NEEDS TO KNOW?

I mentioned earlier the need to tell your close co-workers. They need to know what is happening as soon as possible, even if you do not consider them close friends. Some people might feel strange taking such a personal matter to people they work with, but it has to be done. Hopefully, you have developed a good working relationship with them so you can feel comfortable talking about it. They should know right away so they can start planning to have backup help while you are out of the office assisting your wife.

I calculated 129 hours of sick leave that I took off the first calendar year after diagnosis. That worked out to roughly 16 working days. This time was solely spent caring for my wife and didn't include sick leave for me or any other member of my family.

HUMAN RESOURCES

At first I was worried that I could lose my job because of all the time off. However, I was reassured by my company's HR department that there were laws protecting employees when they or their immediate family members have a life-threatening illness or emergency. They explained all of the options of how I could effectively structure my time off within payroll policies.

They also provided me with local professionals and companies that were able to assist me with all sorts of services. If you work for a large corporation, they are more familiar with the needs of employees who face these events. Their experience will be very beneficial to you. Most will have recommendations and offer services you don't even think of.

I found my place of employment to be a great strength. They provided words of encouragement, emails, and cards, as well as some much needed financial help. This really endeared my company to me and enabled me to reach out to others at work that might be experiencing similar situations.

YIN AND YANG OF WORK

Some days will be harder than others to come into work. It seemed like my focus just wasn't there. On days my wife had an appointment right in the middle of the day, it was hard to come back into work and pick up where I had left off. You will just have to manage that as best you can. You might request, or even be given, a lighter workload during this time, which can help you accomplish certain tasks without being too taxing.

Other days it might be nice to get back to the routine of work after dealing with all of the responsibilities at home. I found if I was off for an extended period of time, my focus upon returning was amazing. If you can't work from home, hopefully you will have some good friends or close family members that will offer to stay with her when you have to go into the office.

WORK FROM HOME

If you are fortunate enough to have a job that will allow you to work from home, I highly recommend this. Your wife will be more comfortable having you there to assist her and this will show your employer that you are trying to balance what you can.

My employer was able to get me remote Internet access, which was a great benefit. It was rather easy for me to take care of emails or conference calls while she was resting.

The bottom line is to focus on your responsibilities as a husband first, then factor in your workload. If you are solely preoccupied with work, it will really affect your ability to give her support. Try to work out this balance as soon as possible.

HER JOB

If your wife works, you will want to get her employer's email so you can keep them up-to-date on her progress. Some of the husbands, whose wives worked from home while recovering, mentioned the need to step in if your wife is accepting too much responsibility. She might paint a prettier picture to her employer, who will naturally be inclined to increase her workload, so your perspective is important.

Your wife might feel guilty leaving her employer in such a predicament and fear losing her job. But again, there are laws that will protect her position, such as The Family and Medical Leave Act (FLMA). Do some research on this so you know your rights, as it will give both of you peace of mind.

If, for whatever reason, you are at odds with either of your places of employment, do not hesitate to look into the laws that protect you. Most of the hospitals and clinics, as well as the literature you will receive, will have helpful information.

Hopefully, it will never have to come to this because you will have enough on your plate without worrying about employment status.

CHAPTER THIRTEEN

Long Term

It will be a long haul. There is no doubt about it!

No matter how much you just want to forget what has happened and move on, cancer will be an ongoing reality for you.

LIFETIME OF MONITORING

In most cases, your wife will have a lifetime of close monitoring, increased testing, and, in some cases, multiple years of cancer treatments. For instance, my wife had an additional five years of hormone treatment using a drug called Tamoxifen for her type of breast cancer. She just wanted to move on and forget about it.

At different times, you may have the opportunity to play the role of food czar, psychologist, psychiatrist, family social worker, and nurse, as I did. If you find yourself having to wear these hats, look at the glass as half full as you move forward.

Food Czar

If old eating habits were nutritionally inadequate, as Food Czar, do not allow the family to revert back to them. Hopefully, your bad eating habits will have been corrected, and you can maintain healthy food choices in your family's daily routine.

As I mentioned earlier, when your wife's appetite returns she will want to eat all of the foods she hasn't been able to. Try to help her limit meals of pizza, burgers, and fried chicken to once a week instead of once a day.

This will probably be the toughest thing you have to tactfully accomplish, but it will be up to you if you notice your wife returning to those habits.

If she quit smoking or gave up other detrimental addictions while going through this, join her. You are a team and what's good for one is good for the other. Encourage healthy, life-long habits to continue.

Psychologist

As the Psychologist, you will have to help your wife with any mental health issues that can be the result of her treatments.

You might have to help her through panic attacks that she might get while driving past the hospitals and clinics where she was treated. The mere thought of it can make her nauseated and light-headed, a response called anticipatory nausea.

Sometimes the mere mention of what she had to go through can trigger these responses. Talk of the positives and do not dwell on the negatives when telling others of her experiences in her presence.

COGNITIVE FUNCTION

Many studies on the cognitive effects of chemotherapy will mention the terms chemo brain or "chemonesia." These drugs can really affect functions of thinking, remembering, and learning.

You may have to remind your wife of what she needs to do and where she needs to be. This can be frustrating for you because you probably relied on her to remind you! Make a mental note or write down what she tells you to help her remember. Jot it down on a calendar so she can check it often.

CONFIDENCE

Your wife may have been confident and outgoing prior to this experience, but now may be fearful of going out in public. After avoiding others during much of her treatments, due to a compromised immune system, you can see how this might happen.

Another reason could be the physical toll taken. It took a lot of prodding to get my wife to go out without a hat, even after her hair started coming in. It took her time to get used to the short curly hairstyle, but once she did, the positive comments she received lifted her spirits and built her self-confidence.

Let her take time in getting back into the social aspect of life. She might feel like a fish out of water at first. Do not try to force her into public situations until she feels ready. If it was something she liked to do prior to her cancer, make sure she eventually takes that step. Getting her prepared for this is a fine line, one you will learn to carefully walk.

Psychiatrist

As a Psychiatrist, you will need to make sure your wife is behaving normally. As her husband, you should have the added advantage of knowing what "normal" is.

Most men can tell when it is "that time of month" for their wife. They will also remember how their wife acted during pregnancy. Because cancer treatments and medications can really play with her hormone levels, it is likely your wife will experience some of the same emotional extremes associated with pregnancy and menstrual cycles

The ups and downs and mood swings can sometimes be a cause for concern. You will notice rather quickly when they are out of balance and you will need to step in if there are longer periods of depression or anger. It is important that you remain calm and encourage her to talk with her doctor if you or your immediate family is negatively affected by these emotions.

Sometimes she might have to take something that will help her regulate these emotions such as an anti-depressant, anti-anxiety, or other mood-altering medication. If she does have to take something for a while, be sure to inform her doctors of their effectiveness so they can find the right combinations. Be sensitive if she has to take them. Do not refer to them as "crazy pills" or make her feel abnormal.

Family Social Worker

As a Social Worker, you will have to wear all of the above hats while focusing on the well-being of you and your family.

The effects of your wife's cancer on your family may manifest many years down the road. If you try to hide or sugarcoat certain aspects of this experience and your children find out, you will most likely be faced with feelings of betrayal and a loss of trust. Because cancer is such a common disease, the example you set in how you deal with it will be how your children and grandchildren will handle it down the line.

Continue to stay involved and active within the cancer community. You and your family can participate in local charities and cancer awareness activities. The American Cancer Society website can give you plenty of volunteer opportu-

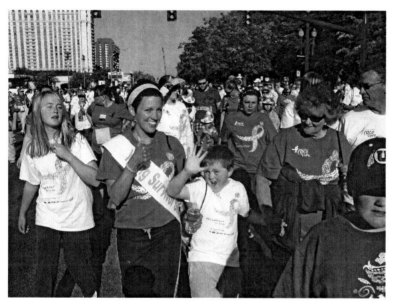

A great day to walk with thousands as we supported Cindy and her mother LaRene as breast cancer survivors.

nities. You don't have to look far to find them. Our family embraced the Race For The Cure run/walk and many other activities to help us deal with it head on.

Nurse

Up to the point of my wife's cancer, I was a big wimp when it came to dealing with blood and family medical situations. I traced this feeling back to my mom being involved in a car accident when I was very young, and I had a hard time visiting her until she was completely healed. Maybe it was just the fear of ever having to deal with injuries or surgeries myself. It has always been hard for me to be able to care for a loved one in distress.

During the birth of our four children, I told the nurses to be prepared to catch me if I faint. The nerves I felt of not being in control, knowing all of the things that could go wrong, and not knowing how I could help if they did, were overwhelming. There was no way I could've ever imagined having to perform nursing duties and feeling comfortable in completing them before this.

This comfort came from having to help take care of her surgical sites for weeks at a time. As with anything in life, the more you do it the better you get.

Having these skills will prepare you for setbacks down the road. A few of these that my wife encountered were incisions opening up soon after surgery, transplanted skin dying due to lack of proper blood supply, implants having to be taken out and put back in, and multiple drains that needed to be emptied and measured.

As I mentioned earlier, you really need to watch what the nurses are doing while you're at the hospital because it is a totally different environment when you get home. Trying to look at a rough "how to" sketch of medical procedures on your discharge papers can be difficult. Having a nurse explain, over the phone, how to do something you should have witnessed firsthand can be confusing as well.

If you work at acquiring these skills, they will better prepare you to handle medical care more professionally and give you "nurses knowledge."

Afterward

I often tell my wife that she is the strongest person I have ever met. She handled her cancer with great resolve and confidence. She made a concerted effort not to let her trial ruin her relationship with our children or me.

I could really tell those days that were just plain awful for my wife, but she remained constant and patient with us. She would often apologize for getting cancer and for the effects she could see it was having on us emotionally, financially, and sometimes spiritually. When she did this, it was a wake-up call for me to change my behavior and try to make sure she did not feel this way.

This journey can be full of setbacks.

A few of my wife's surgeries did not heal correctly, which led to additional surgeries. On one occasion, she had what was called a Latissimus Flap procedure done as part of her breast reconstruction. Within a few weeks, the transplanted skin and muscle began to die. Our doctors could not believe that this happened to someone with such healthy tissue. This led to another surgery called Deep Inferior Epigastric Perforator (DIEP Flap) reconstruction that was a little more evasive. But to my wife's credit, she did not get angry or blame anyone. She accepted the outcome and moved on.

The drug that she took to keep her hormone receptors low led to menopausal symptoms. She would have incredible hot flashes and sweats. The smallest things would make her cry or get her frustrated. When this would happen, she would simply go to our bedroom and calmly remove herself from the situation, realizing that it was the drug's effect on her.

That is basically the attitude you and your wife have to take when dealing with cancer. Not too high and not too low. Do your best to just get through whatever is thrown at you.

One who gains strength by overcoming obstacles possesses the only strength which can overcome adversity. —*Albert Schweitzer*

As good as life can be, it will be full of battles. We both realized this was a major battle.

I felt as if we were two soldiers on the front-line fighting the cancer together. Just as you wouldn't leave a wounded soldier behind, you shouldn't leave your wife behind

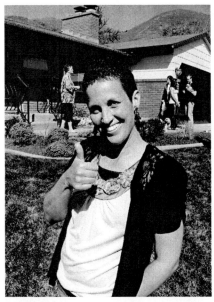

It was a long road but Cindy made it through her chemo and radiation therapy.

when she needs you most. You will have to carry your wife for a while, but it will only make you stronger.

It is my hope and prayer that you both come out of this battle *together*. Strengthened and unified.

You will get through this!

Personal Stories

A few husbands that I reached out to for support accepted the invitation to share some of their feelings and experiences. These stories are both profound and tragic. The point is to help you understand that you are not alone and that others are experiencing similar challenges. Each story is told from the husband's point of view.

KEVIN JOHNSON

Prior to my wife's cancer diagnosis, the only person in my immediate family that had cancer was my paternal grandmother. She was diagnosed with stomach cancer. I was twenty-one years old when I learned that my grandmother's illness was terminal, and there was nothing they could do for her. They brought a hospital bed into her living room at home, and my family and I took turns taking care of her.

The cancer kept eating away until she succumbed to the horrible illness.

My wife was diagnosed with tongue cancer called Squamous cell carcinoma . After beginning treatment, they found she simultaneously had Thyroid cancer, so the doctors had to treat both at the same time.

The cancer started with a burning canker sore that wouldn't heal. My wife was worried that it kept lingering, so she had the dentist look at it first. The dentist wasn't sure what it was and indicated that he hadn't seen anything like it. He referred her to an oral surgeon, who had never seen anything like it, and, therefore, didn't want to even take a biopsy. We then met with our family doctor with the same results. The oral surgeon had recommended that my wife see someone at the Huntsman Cancer Institute in Salt Lake City. We made an appointment with an ear, nose, and throat specialist there. The specialist did a punch biopsy, which came back with negative results. We were relieved and believed that everything was going to be all right.

During this exam, however, some nodules on her thyroid were discovered, so he mentioned he would keep an eye on those. One option he offered was to remove the growth on her tongue so they could find out exactly what it was. We elected to have the surgery done to make sure and he successfully removed the growth. It was out-patient surgery and everything went smoothly. A week later, she went in for the follow-up and official results, which I could not attend because of work conflictions. I decided that I could miss this appointment because things had gone so well with the surgery and the initial test had come back negative. My wife had her mom go with her instead. That afternoon I got the call at work that they had done pathology tests on the growth and it had come back as cancer. They mentioned it was an extremely aggressive and dangerous form of mouth cancer and I felt guilty because I was not there.

This diagnosis led to the removal of margins around the tongue and some lymph nodes to test for spreading of the cancer. Also, while part of the thyroid was removed and quickly tested. The quick test came back positive, so the physicians ended up removing it while they were in there. My wife's hospital stay was five nights combined with a Radioactive iodine treatment, which was tedious and unusual.

After these surgeries and treatments, everything seemed so insignificant. My emotional response was that this was something that happens to other people and it was hard to get my arms around. It was the same feeling I had when my wife and I were told we were going to have premature twins. This was supposed to happen to others. A real dose of reality sets in when you realize you are those other people. There's a lot of fear and anxiety when you don't know what is happening or needs to happen to get rid of the cancer.

Conversations early on, when uncertainty for the future prevailed, led to a decision to not tell many people because we didn't think it was worth worrying other people and assuming the worst. From the beginning, we decided to assume the best and everything would be fine. Initially we were told that it wasn't cancerous and we felt good about not alarming everyone and planned for the best. The shock soon set in when we found out it was cancerous. At that time we felt we needed everyone's positive thoughts and prayers, so we made the conscious decision to tell everybody we could. I spent the whole night on the phone to let everyone know. We still made the decision that no matter what, we were going to plan for the best and tried really hard never to dwell on the negative. The advice I would give to others is that it doesn't do any good to worry about the worst. Your positive energy, positive thoughts, and planning and hoping for the best are the only ways to get through it. If the diagnosis turns out differently, then you can deal with the next steps the same way. The alternative is to be negative, worry, and waste energy on something you can't control. We could have wasted five weeks in the negative alternative from her first surgery until her larger surgery, but it would have done us no good.

I think my wife and I owned the cancer together. It was my wife's illness, but I felt like we needed to face it together. I decided early on that I was going to be with her every step of the way and make sure she knew she had my support. I also wanted to make sure we were being thorough, asking the right questions, and understanding all of our options. In this manner, when we prayed and looked for inspiration, we could identify what direction to go with her treatment plan and then trust that decision. It's important to own the illness and face it together.

As she recovered, I was used to preparing meals. I learned to cook from an early age, but it definitely opens your eyes to how much your wife does for you and your family in so many other areas. It was good for our family to step in and try to help more. I felt these were insignificant duties to have to deal with compared to what she had to deal with and endure. When I thought about it in that way, it was hard to feel sorry for myself. Our children were really good at helping with household chores and they could see how helpless their mother was for long stretches of time. They did a great job helping out.

Our children were between ten and nineteen years old at the time. What my wife and I tried to do was to focus on the positive and give the children the facts. As we talked with them, we told them about the treatment plan, what we expected to happen, and decided not to dwell on the negative. For the most part, all of our children were very positive about it. I think they could sense and see how we were dealing with it, which helped them to remain calm. To have to deal with adversity like this seemed to draw us closer together as a family.

My work and the team I work with were phenomenal in allowing me as much time as I needed. Other than that one appointment when she received her diagnoses, I have not missed one since. Coworkers confirmed that everything I was doing, as far as work was concerned, was insignificant compared to my wife's and family's well-being. They would constantly ask how things were going and if we needed anything. They, along with our neighbors, were fantastic and would bring food and meals over all of the time. Some people did not know how to deal with it and were a little hesitant. But, for the most part, everyone was very thoughtful and giving of their time and in sharing their experiences. I was surprised at how many people have had to deal with cancer. Some of them became our good friends from sharing in such an experience. My wife had one good friend that pulled back for a while, but soon came back around.

Financially, I had great benefits, so we were not as negatively impacted as we could have been, like some other people are. Most employers are facing increasing costs so benefits are being cut, it seems like every year. We were fortunate to have some basic co-pays, which came out-of-pocket, and everything else was taken care of.

My wife and I were extremely grateful for the team of doctors that worked on her. We were fortunate to have a cancer specialist fairly close by because it was a unique cancer for someone that didn't smoke, drink, or chew tobacco. We were told that this type of cancer just didn't occur in people that did not have that type of lifestyle. I wanted to make sure we were going to a physician that dealt with that type of cancer for my peace of mind.

I learned that you never think it is going to happen to you, so you aren't as diligent in taking care of yourself, eating right, and exercising. Something like this opens your eyes and you realize you are as vulnerable as anybody. As important as it is to eat well, exercise, and get sleep, it is also important to get your screenings and checkups done. You need to be aware of changes in your body, as well as your wife's body.

This experience definitely brought us closer together and we learned to value our time together. On the physical side, not being able to kiss her for long stretches of time was very difficult, but it made it all the sweeter when we could do those things again to realize what we had missed. There are a lot of things you take for granted in a relationship. Realizing that really helped in strengthening both of us for whatever lies ahead in the future. I became more tender and nurturing, which are sides I didn't know I had. I had to make sure she took all of her pills and I learned how to be very attentive to her needs. I was able to recognize them before she expressed them.

Cancer can happen to anyone and dealing with it in a positive way, as much as possible, is something you will have to work at. Get a game plan as quick as you can and deal with setbacks as they come. Have a positive outlook, no matter the diagnosis and you will be better for it.

BRAD MORRIS

To begin, my mother had passed away from Multiple Myeloma that she had years prior to me getting married. When we were dating, my future wife would go over and attend to my mother with some of her therapies, as we were both nursing students at the time. Other than this experience with my mother, there was no other history of cancer in my family.

Just before our second anniversary, my wife and I were on a family boating trip and she took a hard fall water skiing, which caused some pain in her belly. When we returned home a few days later, this pain persisted. Some of the symptoms seemed similar to gall bladder disease (which both of us were a little familiar with) so we wondered if this was the case. We ended up going to the emergency room and, at age twenty-three, my wife was diagnosed with a large tumor on one of her ovaries accompanied by free fluid in the pelvis.

After this visit, we set up her surgery with a gynecological oncologist. He planned on removing the tumor because of the size, but all along suspected it was a benign ovarian cyst, which was common in young females. During this surgery, with my wife asleep on the operating table, the doctor came into the waiting room and told me that the frozen section from the tumor tested came back positive.

It was a moment I will never forget!

Sitting there, having the doctor tell my mother-in-law and me that it was positive for *cancer* was horrible!

The doctor then explained the routine was to perform a hysterectomy, remove the ovaries and uterus, and take many more samples to determine the cancer stage. This would help determine the spread of the disease. My mother-in-law was sitting next to me, sort of nodding her head in agreement. I looked at him and said "You know what, we don't have children yet, and I don't know if I should make this decision without her."

I asked him to end the surgery right then, and close her up so I could talk to her and plan together what we should to do next. He agreed and did exactly that. My mother-in-law turned to me after the physician left and commented that she would never have had the courage to recommend that course of action. One thing I learned that day was there is no reason to make rash decisions when it comes to moments like this. You might as well take a few days to really sort out things you really want to do. It takes a few days to get back the official pathology to know exactly what you're dealing with anyway. If I had made the decision to just go with what is the routine, we wouldn't have our four children today.

I was so shocked when I received the diagnosis from the doctor. You have to put your trust in them. When you're told a growth is probably benign and then it's not, it can really be shocking. That was definitely the first emotion to surface for me. The hardest thing I had to do was tell my wife when she woke up that she had cancer. I don't think most doctors feel remotely comfortable giving that news, let alone a husband telling their wife. Once we decided to wait and get the staging results, we were better able to make the determination to do less drastic surgeries and treatments to give ourselves a chance to have a family.

About four weeks later, even though the tumor and ovary were removed during the first operation, we went in for surgery to determine the final stage of the cancer. We also met with the medical oncologist at this time. Chemotherapy was recommended, with close monitoring for the next five to ten years.

She staged low at a 1c out of 4, so her risk statistically for the return of that type of cancer was really low. It was important for us that she made the choice and that our doctor supported her decision. Luckily, that is what happened.

We were not finished, however.

My wife's ovarian cancer resurfaced about ten years later, even though it was a different type than the first go round. This necessitated some further discussion on doing some other tests to determine if she was predisposed to some other cancers or had genetic abnormalities that were causing it. The Breast Cancer (BRCA) genetic test and a few other tests were performed to see if there was a family history link to her cancers. These all came back clear. This time the decision was easy for her to have the hysterectomy, due to the fact we were done having children and the remaining ovary was affected. The staging came back at 1c again and the treatment was similar. The first time she endured six rounds of chemotherapy. This time there were three rounds.

Our four children were all under the age of ten. We had a family conference and I broke the news and told them what was going to happen over the next several weeks. Taking the opportunity to explain my wife's history with cancer early on prepared them for this second battle and made them more attentive to her needs. Preparing them for the hair loss from the chemotherapy was made easier with me shaving my head, as well as our son. We stressed that life really wasn't going to change, and, although there would be hair loss, surgeries, and recovery, they would still go on with their schoolwork and activities.

I used my FMLA (Family and Medical Leave Act) leave when I needed to be home to help take care of my wife and the children. The majority of care came from her parents, her sisters, and a few of my siblings, which was a huge comfort. Some great neighbors helped shuttle the children around. Generally speaking, the second time around my wife tolerated the treatments a lot better than the first time. Part of that, I'm sure, was her doing half as many treatments. She would feel pretty crummy a few days after the chemotherapy, and was generally weak for a few weeks, but she could continue to do the majority of what she usually did, which was very impressive.

My work associates and company were really great. I didn't run into any issues. This time I had enrolled in my companies FLMA program, just in case we ever had to go through cancer again. I had up to twelve weeks I could take off without it affecting my job status, similar to paternity leave. I had colleagues pick up my shifts so I didn't need to use all of it. If I had needed to take off more work, they all said they would be there for me, which was a nice luxury.

My wife did most of the notifying of family and friends because she is the social butterfly and was very open to sharing her whole experience with our Facebook friends. We both shared in getting the word out to our families, however. I have a Facebook account that is run by her, so she also got the word out. I was amazed at how quickly the word spread and the support we received. The only one that really had a hard time with either of her episodes was a sister. No one in her family had any history with cancer, so it was new for her family.

Emotionally, it was a lot easier the second time around because I had dealt with the ups and downs before. Most people thought I was very stoic the first go round and a little bit guarded. I had to keep reminding myself that this was just a trial we would have to go through. My expectation was a full recovery and we would go on. My faith was also paramount in keeping me positive and looking for a positive outcome. At first, it was frustrating how many people came out of the woodwork that wanted to help, and how difficult it was to accept. I soon learned that others needed to provide service and I needed to accept it. It was my wife's battle, but the more we could show support, the easier it would be for her. Even if it is something you don't feel like you need, it's what they need.

Personally for me, my wife's cancer didn't really change me physically because I tried to keep my same routine as before. I continued to stay active and do those things we enjoyed doing as a family. I found by keeping my children on their schedule helped me in keeping with my schedule. We took the children on a trip to Disneyland during her treatments the second time, which gave the children some positive memories from this time. Earlier, we did a multiple week trip to Europe after her first bout, so we really tried to keep doing things we liked to do.

Emotionally, however, the whole experience forced me to have some uncomfortable channels of communication with my wife that you hope you would never have to share. We always kept our feelings close to the vest. Both of us really didn't share a lot of our deep emotions. To have to discuss death so early on in our marriage really strengthened us for future trials. We are both more open in sharing our feelings about life and our experiences together and with others.

In most cases, there is no reason to rush through the process of treatments, choosing a surgeon, and radical surgeries. Take your time to find the right team, the right scenario, making the right decision, and pursuing the right plan. I think that is pivotal. Knowing you can put your trust in the medical team and they can put their trust in you is important in moving forward together.

It is really easy, when you're told your wife has cancer, to get in to a doctor right away and get it taken care of immediately. Taking the time to find the right team of doctors is critical. Depending on the stage, if it is caught early, there is time and you don't need to rush to judgment on a treatment course.

I would also add that I wish we had looked into life insurance for my wife earlier in our marriage, especially since most companies will not let you get it for five to ten years after her recovery. If there is a history of cancer on either side of her family, the sooner you can get a policy in place the less expensive it will be.

BRENT BOVERO

I was seven or eight years old when my paternal grandfather died of cancer in California. I remember my dad being very upset, but not really understanding what he had or what had happened. About five years later, my maternal grandfather died of cancer as well. I can remember my parents being upset about it, but not really communicating to us children the specifics or what kind of cancer it was.

Years later, I was married with a couple of small children when my mother came over to visit one evening. I noticed that she started to look a little bloated. We talked her into visiting the doctor, even though she hated doctor's visits, and it we soon discovered that she had breast cancer. This was the mid-70s and my mother had never really gone in to have the lump checked, so by the time they could check it, it was a stage four cancer. I remember thinking at the time that this kind of thing happens to other people's parents, but not mine. They were only in their late fifties at the time, and I figured they had at least another ten to fifteen years of good health. I just couldn't imagine being without my parents.

We would visit my mother at the hospital after they had done a radical mastectomy and she was there for a few weeks. She would try to chuckle at each visit to lessen the severity of her situation. Many times she would become so bloated she would have to go into the hospital to have the pressure released from her stomach area. During one of these visits, I was informed she was not doing well and to get there quickly. I showed up as soon as I could from work, hoping to see my mom before she passed away. When I arrived, I found myself alone with her in her hospital room. All of the instruments and monitoring devices had been rolled up and it hit me hard that she was gone. My dad and siblings were waiting in another room. It was about nine to ten months after she was diagnosed that she passed away. After the experience with my mother, cancer became a bad word for me because I believed there really wasn't anything positive that could come from it.

A few years later, my brother came to me asking questions about what my bleeding ulcers I had growing up felt like and what some of the symptoms were. I told him and his experiences seemed similar, so he thought he had the same thing. He started taking over-the-counter antacids that seemed to work for a while. Then, while on a trip, he was cooking some steaks when he was in so much pain he couldn't even eat and came straight home to see a doctor about it. He went in, and when I got to the hospital to check on him, my sister informed me that it was Stomach Cancer in the lining of the walls. He only lived a few months after that, and I watched him gradually wither away. He went from a healthy 210 pounds down to about 75 pounds by the time he died. I began to feel that cancer was haunting my side of the family. A few years prior to my brother's death, his son had died of the same form of stomach cancer at the age of twenty-one.

In addition to my mother passing away due to breast cancer, her sister, my aunt, had passed away from it also. Then her daughter, my cousin, had breast cancer as well, but she was able to beat hers. She was the first positive outcome of cancer in my family up to this point.

Then it started to enter into my own family when my daughter was diagnosed with breast cancer in her thirties. I figured her cancer must have been a connection through my side of the family because my wife's history of cancer contained only one uncle that had cancer.

It was during my daughter's recovery from her mastectomies that my wife went in for her annual mammogram. It was standard practice for her to go in every year and within a few days they would call and say everything looked good. This time we got the call from the hospital asking for my wife and wanting her to call back. After I hung up, I got thinking why they didn't just tell me everything is all right. I started to worry a little bit.

My wife went back in to have the mammogram performed a second time. They noticed what they thought was a smudge on the mammogram, so she went back in for another one as well as an ultrasound. They then brought the charts in from the previous year to show her the differences between the two images. I was not with her during these first few appointments because I thought they screwed up with the first one and everything would be all right. I still had doubts coming to my mind. A few days later, they wanted her to go in for a biopsy. I didn't go to that one as well because I assumed this was routine. I was putting in a fence at the time and thought nothing of it because she had no history of cancer on her side of the family.

A few days later our family doctor called and wanted to see both of us in person, which was unusual as I expected a phone call saying everything would be all right. When our family doctor told us it was Invasive Ductal Carcinoma, the same type of cancer my daughter had, I could hardly believe it. They showed us the picture and how small it was.

They explained that they could probably remove it with a procedure called a lumpectomy.

We then met with a few different teams of doctors, but ended up settling on the same doctors that my daughter had worked with. We went in for the procedure. Everything went really well and the doctors said she did great. About a week later, we went up for her checkup and they went over the pathology report and said that all of the margins were clear except for one microscopic area. A few days later we were back in for a quick procedure to get a larger margin. We found out her tumor was almost two centimeters in size, which was a lot bigger than initially diagnosed. They decided to take a few lymph nodes to make sure it wasn't on the move. She also had what was called an Oncotype DX test (ONCA) to help determine what she should do as far as treatments were concerned. Because she was on the border of the recommendations on this test due to the tumor size, it was left up to us to decide.

Some of the doctors we met with recommended chemotherapy, and others radiation with mastectomy. Needless to say, my wife and I were very confused at what she should do. Our daughter had chemotherapy, double mastectomy, and radiation, so we didn't know if she needed all of that as well. I remember having a hard time concentrating on anything during this time because it was so hard to focus. It was always three more days, or six more days, or ten more days and we'll know what to do. This seemed to go on for months. We both wanted to be told what she should do, but it was left up to us.

We really started reaching out to friends who had dealt with her type of cancer and similar size tumor to see what they had done. We also talked with our daughter. Because her hormone receptors had come back positive, my wife finally made the decision to do a mastectomy with a five-year chemotherapy treatment of a drug called Tamoxifen. We were grateful that the cancer had not spread to her lymph nodes. It was a great relief when she decided on a plan of action.

If I had one recommendation, it would be to watch what the nurses are doing with the surgery site after any operations. If you don't, you might have a hard time following paper explanations and having to take instructions over the phone. Watching and asking questions while they are doing it is a must. For instance, my wife had some drain tubes that I would have to help her drain and I was stretching the tube improperly at first, which would cause my wife needless pain. I learned really fast how to do it properly, but I felt embarrassed that I didn't do it right the first few times.

The whole experience was such a roller coaster for me. I started to think about my age, how much time I have left, and what is important and what is not important. Sometimes, I would lose my motivation on certain projects I wanted to do. I also didn't have a desire to play softball during this time, which was something I always enjoyed. I felt like I aged a few years in just a four-month timeframe. I really hated nighttime because I had a hard enough time sleeping after I retired, but after my daughter and then my wife were going through this, I could not get negative thoughts out of my mind. I would be lucky if I got an hour or two of good sleep. I kept thinking two years ago none of this was in my own family. I always felt I would be the one to get cancer in behalf of my family and a burden I would have to bare.

I still struggle with negative thoughts from time to time, but I found by reaching out to others and seeing how positive they were in handling their cancer made me feel that there is no benefit to let it affect me in such a negative manner. My wife has always been the strong one in the relationship. I can get ornery now and again, but I also can wear my emotions on my sleeve. I can handle pain, but emotionally I have a harder time controlling it. My wife and daughter were so strong and I felt so bad that I couldn't take on the burden for them, but I could do my best to help them wherever possible.

I have never been the most religious person because my parents were never really active in their religion, which explains why I'm sort of off and on as well. When something like this happens, it really drives you to prayer and having faith that things will work out for the best.

When I saw how hard my wife worked and helped out with our daughter and her family, and then would come home and keep everything going, it really made me respect and appreciate all that she does for me. To have three surgeries in a matter of months, and then to deal with it with such perseverance and patience, was amazing. Even when she was in pain, she would just keep going.

Those that will have to deal with cancer have my deepest sympathy and my utmost respect. I've learned to never back down from talking with people and sharing my experience. Have faith in the doctors and the treatments that will be administered. Don't let it eat you completely inside and dwell on it twenty-four hours a day. Once the shock of it subsides, get a plan together and reach out to others. You do not have to deal with this by yourself. Get as many first-hand experiences as you can from those you know and trust. Avoid the second- or third-hand accounts because they might not have the information you will need. No matter what, stay positive and stay active in this process and you can get through it together.

KENT GODFREY

Personally, I had never had to deal with cancer too closely. On my side of the family, no one had ever had cancer. On my wife's side, her grandma and aunt each had breast cancer twice. Both of them passed away after we were married. I also remember a girl in high school had died of cancer, but I didn't know what type.

My wife had just turned forty and we were changing health insurance programs, so my wife decided to have her first mammogram on our old plan. After her results came back, the doctor said there was something unusual and wanted her to come back in for another screening. We both thought that was strange, but this being her first mammogram we thought maybe this was a common occurrence.

After the second mammogram, the doctors said the strange mass was still there and they wanted to biopsy it. I went with my wife to this appointment where they took the sample and had it tested. This is when we found out it was a form of breast cancer called Ductal Carcinoma in Situ (DCIS). I started to worry about what we were going to do next and my wife cried a little bit. A consultation with the doctors provided information for what doctors we needed to visit and possible tests and treatment options that might be involved with her type of cancer. Because we were receiving the information from the mammogram doctors and not cancer specialists, we were overwhelmed. The nurse assured us that my wife would be fine, but cancer was cancer to me.

When my wife and I arrived home, we told our children that we had received some pictures from the doctor that showed that their mom had a form of breast cancer and she was about to go through some surgeries and treatments. Our two youngest children started to cry. Our oldest son sat speechless, but our next oldest son simply asked if mom was going to die? He was fine after we reassured him that she was not going to die. We had to do some major consoling and reassuring with the younger ones. They wanted their mom no matter what, whether she was sick or not, and they really didn't comprehend what was going on at first.

My wife and I then informed my wife's parents, my parents, and the rest of our family. Additionally, we told a few people at church and the word started to spread fast from there. My wife really didn't like being the center of attention and she mentioned to everyone to not tell that many people. Our children didn't listen and did a good job of spreading the word to their teachers and friends at school, so the circle of those that knew grew quickly. At work I told a few close associates, but that was all because I didn't want it going around the office to people I really didn't know.

I'm the kind of guy that plans for the worst sometimes, so not knowing what was next was very painful. I tried to plan for the best, but it was pretty shocking and kind of made my world stop. Once the initial shock passed after a couple of weeks, it was very helpful for me that most everyone knew. However, a lot of people would comment to me that they knew someone who had it and that they were just fine, so they were sure my wife would be fine. A lot of them really didn't know how to act and tried to avoid talking about it. I guess I was looking for more sympathy, but I figured it was their way of showing support.

After my wife and I met with the a few different oncologist doctors at different hospitals, we felt good working with a hospital that specializes in just cancer. Because it was pre-cancer, my wife settled on a lumpectomy procedure to remove the suspect tissue. It was determined during these early visits that she did not need to have radiation or chemotherapy. In fact, the first surgery went so well we were able to go camping the next day, which surprised me.

The doctors recommended that she have some genetic testing done due to her family history of breast cancer. She was given the BRCA (Breast Cancer) test and it came back positive, so her percentages of the breast cancer returning, as well as ovarian cancer, were pretty high. This news led her to do a double mastectomy and have her ovaries removed. She was in surgery for eight hours to complete all of the surgeries and tests. This procedure took her a few weeks to bounce back from.

I found from this experience that cancer treatment is a process and the final results come much later. For instance, if you have appendicitis they simply go in and remove the appendix, but with cancer it seems like they start small and then get more drastic depending on each stage of the results. After the mastectomy, they went through the tissue and realized it had started to spread, so it really was Invasive Ductal Carcinoma. Had we just stayed with the lumpectomy, the doctors figured radiation would have kept it from spreading, but we were both glad all of the tissue was taken out and studied. To be told she had DCIS, and then to find out it was on the move, shows you that cancer identification is a process and not a quick result. Had my wife's BRCA come back negative, they would have just done radiation.

I recommend meeting with a genetic counselor if your wife's genetic testing comes back positive. The knowledge my wife and I learned about what she was predisposed to was very valuable. We learned that there are fifteen steps from birth to cancer, and depending on what genetic variable you have, you might be starting on step six instead of one at birth. We learned that this gene could be passed on to our children. We have four children, so it makes it likely that two have it and two don't. In our boys, it will be very rare that they ever get breast cancer, but they could pass it on to their daughters. Just because my daughter is a carrier does not mean she will get breast cancer, but they will monitor her more closely and likely start checking in her mid-twenties.

My place of employment was on the way to the hospital, so I was able to be there for her appointments. Luckily, my employer worked with me with all of my time off. We also had such good support from family and friends. I realized that cancer is not a death sentence and to remain calm until you have all of the facts of what you are dealing with. If you are not a level-headed person you might have a hard time processing the results. It is important that you get through it and see her through it. There are a lot of horror stories that you might have heard or hear as you go through this, but I decided to dwell on all of the positive stories and studies we received.

My faithful prayers, along with having family and others pray for us really helped. I'm a worrier by nature, but I felt that everything would work out okay. My faith helped keep me calm and my head clear.

Personally, I was pretty stoic through the whole process and felt like I needed to pick up the slack and make sure the children did their part in supporting their mother. I felt we were blessed that she didn't have to go through chemo therapy or radiation, as those treatments could have made it much worse. My wife mentioned that I became very compassionate and tried to make sure she had what was needed during her recoveries.

We both feel like we can count on and appreciate each other more than ever.

LARRY KIRBY

In looking back at my history with cancer, the only person in my family to have cancer was my father. He had prostate cancer very late in his life. He actually died of Alzheimer disease before the cancer had a chance to take him. There was also some minor skin cancer, but no deaths due to it.

When my wife found a lump on the inside of her knee, I had no idea that it would be the beginning of a long cancer battle. She had fallen down the stairs and thought it was a bruise that would go away eventually. When the pain persisted for more than a few days, she went to a local clinic, which didn't know what it was, so they referred her to an orthopedic specialist. The specialist made the comment that it was most likely a Sarcome, which was a very rare and aggressive cancer, and recommended she see a specialist. I was on a fishing trip during this visit. My wife called to tell me what the doctor thought, and I felt awful I wasn't there. All of this happened within a two-week period, and I was in total denial that it could be that serious.

The specialist my wife and I met with was nationally known as one of the best doctors to treat that type of cancer. When the initial biopsy of the growth came back negative, we were very relieved. The doctor wanted to remove it to make sure there was nothing there, so we scheduled surgery to have it taken out. After her surgery, the lump was confirmed to be a stage 3 Sarcoma, and the doctors would have to run many more tests to see if it had spread. I wondered how we went from a negative biopsy to full-blown cancer? Were biopsies even reliable? It was explained to me that the cancerous tumor had a capsule of benign tissue wrapped around it and that is why the initial biopsy came back negative. Once the doctors removed the tumor, they were able to test a full section. I ended up having to tell my wife what it was when she woke up, which was very difficult to do.

I started to panic once I got on the computer and started researching her type and stage of cancer. The information was not very positive. I started dwelling on the survival rate, which was about fifty percent under these scenarios. Sarcomas are hard to cure the first time and they tend to resurface in the same spot or the lungs. My wife was very positive and just let the process take its course. I was more of an emotional mess with all of the information and studies I was reading. I continued to exercise a lot and that seemed to help me because my bad eating habits, especially ice cream, really increased during this time.

It was hard for our three grown daughters to be told this news, but our youngest son, who was in high school at the time, did not want to hear anything about it. The fact that she had cancer was too much for him to hear, and I didn't help the situation when I informed him about the survival statistics. I learned you have to reveal difficult information in stages versus just dumping it on your family all at once. He distanced himself from it all and still won't talk about it today. Be prepared for any reaction, as you never know how your children will deal with news like this. Our daughters are reminded of their mother's cancer whenever they go in for their doctor appointments and are asked if a family member has had cancer. They tell them about their mother and the doctors can get very alarmed, so it is something they will have to deal with the rest of their lives. She had no cancer on her side of the family, so it was hard for her family to deal with it as well.

My wife's surgery was successful and the doctor felt they had removed the tumor with clean margins. She went through multiple radiation treatments that hit that area hard. They began meeting with her every three months to do a CT scan of her mid-section for any sign of tumors. Sure enough, about two years later, a spot developed on her lung. The doctors weren't quite sure it was Sarcoma, so they ended up just watching it for a while because it would require surgery just to biopsy it. About five years from the time of her knee surgery, they decided to operate on her lung and figure out what the spot was. Even though it wasn't growing, it wasn't going away either.

The biopsy of the spot on my wife's lung turned out to be a slow growing Sarcoma and because it had metastasized, it was considered a stage 4 cancer. In fact, it was really close to entering her lymph nodes in her lung. We were both shocked that we were back in the same predicament, but felt fortunate they caught it before it spread further.

My wife's doctor is really great and has a great sense of humor, which really helps. My wife feels so comfortable with him. It is very important that your wife feels at ease around her doctors because they will get to know the physicians very well from all of the visits and the emotional nature of it all. Since I travel a lot for work, I am always worried about attending a lot of her appointments, but I am surprised that with a little planning how many I'm able to attend.

To most of our friends and neighbors, my wife looked fine and healthy on the outside, so they didn't realize the seriousness of what she was dealing with. I understood that she wasn't going through treatments that could change her appearance, but it bothered me that she received very little attention, other than from our children and a few people that really knew what was going on. I recognized that I was being a little selfish, but I wanted her to get more attention than she was.

My wife really didn't get down emotionally until she had her lung surgery. She then had hip replacement surgery a few months later. She was in a lot of pain and discomfort as she went through physical therapy. I was amazed that she was able to come out of it so quickly, however.

The majority of the time, my wife dealt with all of the insurance and hospital payment issues and most of the time it went smoothly. However, make sure you find out if the hospital you're going to work through has their own billing department or if they outsource it to a third party company. One hospital that performed some tests outsourced their billing. The collection company was a very aggressive and started calling about bills that needed to be paid, sometimes before the actual due date. They would threaten us that if we didn't pay it right away it would affect our credit. We couldn't believe how insensitive they were. It takes a while for your insurance company to pay their portion and then let you know what yours is, so avoid these situations if at all possible.

Now, my wife has a lifetime of monitoring her body and if the tumors resurface anywhere, the doctors will have to take them out. I sometimes just want to hear that the cancer is gone and will never come back, but we both realize the reality of the situation. My wife is an inspiration with how upbeat she is and a good example for me on how to face challenges with the right attitude. She was able to overcome her negative thoughts the year she had the two surgeries. She just has the faith that her body can manage the cancer, and have faith in the doctors and technology to make sure they pick up anything in the future.

STEVE COLEMAN

My wife, Tana, was thirty-one years old when she was diagnosed with Stage 3b breast cancer. To say I wasn't prepared for the news would be an understatement. I appreciated speaking with friends and family, and I am grateful for their support. That said, I didn't feel like any of them could truly relate to what Tana and I were going through. I reached out to a friend who had lost his wife to breast cancer and I felt like he understood what I was going through. He had credibility when he answered my questions. I found other breast cancer husbands who became great friends and resources through the process. Through the years, I have had the opportunity to speak with other husbands about their sweetheart being diagnosed with cancer. It has been very healing for me to answer their questions. You can feel free to reach out to me at colemansb@gmail.com if you would like to speak with a breast cancer husband.

The key for me was to make sure Tana felt comfortable through the process of choosing an oncologist, surgeon, plastic surgeon, chemo site, radiology site, hospital, and surgery center. I supported her in creating her plan and then supported that plan. From diagnosis—choosing physicians, chemo, mastectomy (if needed), radiation (if needed), reconstruction (if needed)—and through follow-up, many friends and family tried to interject their own opinions and agenda. My job was to make sure my sweet wife had time to heal and that other people understood we welcomed their love and support, but had already created a plan.

Please focus on taking care of your wife, your children, and yourself. Your wife and you only have so much time in a day, and every waking minute should be in line with your plan. Be compliant with your treatment parameters, and do not bring any extra stress into your lives. Everyone who will offer support has great intentions and wants to help you and your wife. That said, there is a tendency for some people to make helping your wife more about themselves and less about your wife. Family members and friends mean well, but it is imperative that you act as a gate-keeper and only let those around your wife who truly need to be around her. It is not your responsibility, nor do you have the time, to carry others through the journey you are about to take.

Tana wanted to make chemo "fun." She did a great job of making herself and others feel as happy as possible during chemo treatments. I have to admit I was reluctant, but grabbed on with both hands and supported her in her efforts to organize activities at the chemo unit during all of our sessions. It made chemo a little easier on her and the other patients who were in the unit appreciated the activities we held during treatment.

Tana reached out to a few young survivors and became one of the first ten members in a Young Survivor Sisters support group. I was reluctant to attend the functions and activities, but did so with a smile. Supporting her desire to be part of this group made her happy and helped us make some lifelong friends. Attending Susan G Komen's Race For The Cure was a huge boost for my wife. If your wife wants to go . . . Go!

This may sound crazy, but be grateful for what you are about to go through. The "through sickness and in health" part of your wedding vow was no joke! Now man up and hold up to your vow! Holding her hand while bad news is given, shaving her head so she felt in control, cleaning up after chemo sickness, staying attracted to her throughout the surgery process, and being the gatekeeper to her treatment is one of the greatest things I have had the privilege to experience in my life. Tana and I are closer because of what we have been through. I am grateful for the opportunity I had to battle with her and to serve her.

Checklist

- Review your experience with cancer and how it has affected you.
- Recognize and deal with the shock and fear.
- Learn as much as you can about your wife's type of cancer.
- Tell everyone you can think of that should know.
    - *Family*
    - *Friends*
    - *Co-workers*
    - *Neighbors*
    - *Ecclesiastical leaders*
- Settle on the doctors.
    - *General Surgeon*
    - *Plastic Surgeon*
    - *Medical Oncologist*
    - *Radial Oncologist*
    - *Other*
- Identify *your* responsibilities and identify those that will assist you with:
    - *Children*
    - *Meals*
    - *Appointments*
    - *Household chores*
    - *Other*

- Familiarize yourself with household chores and how and when to do them.
  - *Laundry*
  - *Shopping*
  - *Cooking*
  - *Other*
- Figure the costs and how they are going to be paid.
  - *Insurance coverage*
  - *Financial assistance*
  - *One time payment benefit*
  - *Fund raisers*
  - *Other*
- Recognize other detrimental emotions and how you will deal with them.
  - *Depression*
  - *Anxiety*
  - *Anger and Resentment*
  - *Jealousy*
  - *Paranoia*
  - *Other*
- Get acquainted with ways to increase attentive behavior and demonstrate sensitivity.
- Implement a plan to improve your health and well being.
  - *Exercise*
  - *Healthy diet*
  - *Hobbies*
  - *Spirituality*
  - *Other*

- Customize your work schedule to balance your responsibilities at home and on the job.
- Identify your abilities to wear the different hats in the areas below:
  - *Food Czar*
  - *Psychologist*
  - *Psychiatrist*
  - *Family Social Worker*
  - *Nurse*

Resources

You will want to do a lot of research when your wife has cancer. Here is a list of website resources that I found the most helpful when Cindy had cancer and were used when researching material for this book.

- **American Cancer Society**: www.cancer.org
- **Anticipatory Nausea**: http://motherswithcancer. wordpress.com/2008/06/24/anticipatory-nausea/
- **BRCA Genetic Testing**: http://www.cancer.gov/cancertopics/factsheet/Risk/BRCA
- **Cancer and Sexuality**: http://health.usnews.com/ health-conditions/cancer/information-on-sexuality-and-cancer
- **Cancer Diet Tips**: http://www.helpguide.org/life/ healthy_diet_cancer_prevention.htm
- **Cancer Treatment Centers of America**: www.cancercenter.com
- **Chemo Alopecia**: http://www.mayoclinic.com/health/ hair-loss/CA00037

- **Chemo Brain**: http://www.mayoclinic.com/health/chemo-brain/DS01109
- **Chemotherapy**: http://www.webmd.com/cancer/questions-answers-chemotherapy
- **Cytoxan**: http://www.ncbi.nlm.nih.gov/pubmed-health/PMH0000570/
- **Deep Inferior Epigastric Perforator (DIEP)**: http://www.breastcancer.org/treatment/surgery/reconstruction/types/diep
- **Ductal Carcinoma in Situ (DCIS)**: http://www.mayoclinic.com/health/dcis/DS00983
- **Epirubicin**: http://www.ncbi.nlm.nih.gov/pubmed-health/PMH0000212/
- **Explaining Cancer to Children**: http://www.cancer.org/treatment/childrenandcancer/helpingchildren-whenafamilymemberhascancer/dealingwithdiagnosis/dealing-with-diagnosis-toc
- **Family and Medical Leave Act (FLMA)**: http://www.dol.gov/whd/fmla/
- **Genetic Counseling**: http://www.ornl.gov/sci/techresources/Human_Genome/medicine/genecounseling.shtml
- **HER2 positive test**: http://www.mayoclinic.com/health/breast-cancer/AN00495
- **Huntsman Cancer Institute**: www.huntsmancancer.org
- **Invasive Ductal Carcinoma (IDC)**: http://www.breastcancer.org/symptoms/types/idc

- **Latissimus Flap**: http://emedicine.medscape.com/article/1274087-overview
- **Magnetic Resonance Imaging (MRI)**: http://www.webmd.com/a-to-z-guides/magnetic-resonance-imaging-mri
- **Mammograms**: http://www.cancer.gov/cancertopics/factsheet/detection/mammograms
- **Mayo Clinic**: www.mayoclinic.com
- **Multiple Myeloma**: http://www.cancercenter.com/landing-pages/multiple-myeloma/default.cfm
- **Neupogen**: http://www.ncbi.nlm.nih.gov/pubmed-health/PMH0000912/
- **Oncotype DX test (ONCA)**: http://www.mybreast-cancertreatment.org/en-US/AboutOncotypeDX.aspx?
- **Ovarian Cancer**: http://www.ncbi.nlm.nih.gov/pubmedhealth/PMH0001891/
- **Radioactive Iodine Therapy (Radioiodine)**: http://www.cancer.org/cancer/thyroidcancer/detailedguide/thyroid-cancer-treating-radioactive-iodine
- **Radiation Therapy**: http://www.cancer.gov/cancer-topics/factsheet/Therapy/radiation
- **Sarcoma Cancer**: http://www.cancer.net/cancer-types/sarcoma
- **Scopolamine Patch**: http://www.nlm.nih.gov/medlineplus/druginfo/meds/a682509.html
- **Squamous Cell Carcinoma**: http://www.ncbi.nlm.nih.gov/pubmedhealth/PMH0001832/
- **Stomach Cancer**: http://www.webmd.com/cancer/stomach-gastric-cancer

- **Tamoxifen**: http://www.drugs.com/tamoxifen.html
- **Taxotere**: http://www.ncbi.nlm.nih.gov/pubmed-health/PMH0000987/
- **Thyroid Cancer**: http://www.ncbi.nlm.nih.gov/pubmedhealth/PMH0002193/
- **Total Intravenous Anaesthesia (TIVA)**: http://www.ebme.co.uk/arts/tiva/
- **Young Survivor Sisters blog**: http://youngsurvivor-sisters.blogspot.com/
- **Web MD:** www.webmd.com
- **Women Cancer Statistics:** http://onlinelibrary.wiley.com/store/10.3322/caac.20121/asset/20121_ftp.pdf;jsessionid=5FB64DE0F240E0E06B2D4EF7689FF7D6.d04t04?v=1&t=hesu612p&s=6467f696a996e50e62370a8397825c6c172e51f4

About Carson Boss

Carson Boss is a devoted husband and father who feels blessed to carry both titles. He currently resides in Syracuse, Utah and has lived in Texas and Alberta, Canada. He enjoys singing, performing in Community Theater and traveling around the world meeting new people and experiencing other cultures.

He would love to hear from you and can be reached in the following manner:

Carsonscancercomments@yahoo.com

Carsonscancercomments.blogspot.com

About Familius

Welcome to a place where mothers are celebrated, not compared. Where heart is at the center of our families, and family at the center of our homes. Where boo boos are still kissed, cake beaters are still licked, and mistakes are still okay. Welcome to a place where books—and family—are beautiful. Familius: a book publisher dedicated to helping families be happy.

Familius was founded in 2012 with the intent to align the founders' love of publishing and family with the digital publishing renaissance which occurred simultaneous with the Great Recession. The founders believe that the traditional family is the basic unit of society, and that a society is only as strong as the families that create it.

Familius' mission is to help families be happy. We invite you to participate with us in strengthening your family by being part of the Familius family. Go to www.familius.com to subscribe and receive information about our books, articles, and videos.

Website: www.familius.com
Facebook: www.facebook.com/paterfamilius
Twitter: @familiustalk, @paterfamilius1
Pinterest: www.pinterest.com/familius

CPSIA information can be obtained at www.ICGtesting.com
Printed in the USA
BVOW040336020413

317016BV00002B/17/P